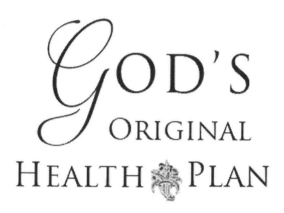

GOD'S
ORIGINAL
HEALTH PLAN

RUBY L. JOHNSON

Publisher:
Ruby L. Johnson, Minister
901-826-2558
rubyjohnson1213@gmail.com

Editing – Dr. Denise Lofton

Stroudmark Photography
901-826-3292
stroudmark@live.com
www.facebook.com/stroudmarkphotography

Created in the United States of America

Warning – Disclaimer
The purpose of this book is to encourage, educate, and
enlighten. Nothing in this book is neither medical nor legal
advice. The author and or publisher do not guarantee that
anyone following the techniques, suggestions, tips, ideas, or
strategies will become successful. The author and publisher shall
have neither liability nor responsibility to anyone with respect to
loss or damage caused, or alleged to be caused, directly or
indirectly by the information contained in this book.

ISBN: 1548865680
ISBN-13: 978-1548865689

DEDICATION

In loving memory of, Rosie L. Hopson, my other grandmother, known as Mama, is the one who reared me. I will always be grateful to her for caring for me. Willie and Pearlie M. Jones, (uncle and aunt), Alberta Crawford, (mother), Rachel Washington (aunt), and Reverend Kenneth T. Whalum, Sr. (former pastor, who was like a father to me and my children), my life was touched by their love.

CONTENTS

Acknowledgments

First, I would like to thank my Heavenly Father who made all this possible. He has been guiding, protecting, and leading me. When I didn't understand much about life, God was there and never left me. I thank my Heavenly Father for giving me wisdom, knowledge and understanding through His Word to write this book.

Edward C Johnson, my husband, who supports me in everything that I do. He is my biggest fan, and my best friend. My beautiful adorable children, they are the world's greatest children: Eddie (Stephanie), Marie, Dennis, and Tina (Maurice), my step children: Edward Jr. (Juanita), Harold, and Adrian. My beautiful grandchildren and great grandchildren; whom I love dearly.

The rest of my wonderful family; my daddy, Mr. Henry L. Dickson, my other mother, Mrs. Prince E. Dickson; uncles, aunts, sisters, brothers, nieces and, nephews, I thank you for your love and support.

My wonderful Pastor, Dr. Kenneth Twigg Whalum Jr., my beautiful First Lady, Mrs. Sheila Whalum, they are authors of several books and my Olive family, thanks for your love and support.

Special Thanks To:

Tammy Adolphus
Debra Cummings
Valerie Wright

PREFACE

HEALTH IS ESSENTIAL

Good health is essential in order to have longevity. This book is designed to encourage people to take a serious look at their health conditions, and what changes need to take place. In today's society, there are so many health problems. By making a few lifestyle changes, you can get on the right track for better health. This book gives you step-by-step instructions how to make those changes. There is something in this book for the entire family.

I was prompted to write this book after dealing with my mother's illness. Her illness made me realized that something was seriously wrong with her health situation. I began to research and gather information along with my knowledge, by visiting different hospitals to generate this book. Also, I sought spiritual guidance from the Word of God.

The answers for your well-being are in this book. I show you through the Word of God, examples through research, and personal experience. I give you examples of those things that will keep you healthy and give you a prosperous life, as well as those that will hinder your life.

1

You might want to eliminate some food items from your list that might be causing major problem. The book is designed to educate people on lifestyle changes. Having good health is so important. When you have good health, you are energetic, happy, excited about life, and a bright future. It explains how you can restore your health through Mother Nature, by eating fruits, vegetables, nuts and grains of the earth. God designed it this way, and He always knows what is best for each of us. It's amazing what a little discipline can do to change your health situation.

Good health is the key to longevity, and if we don't get a handle on the health situation, this society is doomed. You can overcome your health issues by allowing the Word of God to control and direct your life. You can rise above your health circumstances, by giving God control of your health. He wants to help you with every situation you may encounter; therefore, He can certainly help you with your health issues. Give God the opportunity to deliver you from health woes.

INTRODUCTION

I am inspired by God to write this book to help the people of God get a grip on health issues we face in society today. This can be done through utilizing the health plan that God has already put in place. My advice and guidance is grounded in the Word of God and may not agree with the words of man. The world is in a state of confusion due to a lack of knowledge concerning God's Word. You must remember that God is not the author of confusion, but of trust (Psalms 71:1). I must admit that I have never considered myself a writer, but God has taken me to another level (Ask HIM, and He will do the same for you). After coping with my mother's health issues and her death in 2004, my interest in healthy eating became a commitment. Since that time, I have not been able to shake this feeling that I should be doing more, hence, I am writing a book about health matters.

I have been destined by God to dig deeper, to get to the root of our health problems. After seeing so many of God's people plagued with all types of sickness and disease, I decided that it was time for me to educate God's people, according to His Word, concerning our health. So many people have it twisted by believing that diseases are hereditary, and that they are automatically prone to have the same health problems as others in their family. YET, God has requirements for His healing, not the least of which is your belief and your service. In Exodus 23:25 it states, *"And you shall serve the LORD (the eternally self-existing One) your God, and He shall bless thy bread and thy water; and I will take sickness away from the midst of thee."* If you believe, you can reverse generational curses and correct thy path, for generations to come.

When you study God's Word, you will know that sickness and disease are not of God, but of Satan who tries to hinder God's people from serving Him effectively. So many people have become victims and have fallen into Satan's trap and are hindered from serving God (1Thessalonians 2:18). Sickness and disease knows no age limit; all of us may be affected by health issues at some point in our lives. The hospitals are full of ill people young and old, who have been seeking healing from the wrong source ---through man and prescription drugs.

You don't have to have gout, headaches, night sweats, gain weight, or even have heart disease and diabetes. Many common sicknesses can be controlled or cured just by changing our eating habits. As we begin to listen to God's voice through His Word, and not the voice of man, we can seek guidance from the right source, "The Giver of Life". The problem is that we are seeking guidance from the wrong source. For some people, God is some foreign object that is beyond their reach. They seek guidance and trust man to take care of their issues, rather than God. For others, too much emphasis is placed on what man says, rather than what God says, for our life. For example, a person goes to the doctor and is diagnosed with some type of disease (high blood pressure). The first thing the doctor does is to prescribe medication for the rest of your life. Most people never question their doctor nor do they seek advice from God concerning their health issues before going to see a doctor. It appears that most doctors do not take the time to educate their patients on how to change their life style and become healthy again. Emphasis is placed on medications rather than changing that person's life style. According to a magazine article written by Kristin Ohlson, "Physicians annually write nearly 100 million prescriptions for the drugs in the United States, 20 million in England, and 10 million in Canada. In addition, people buy billions of nonprescription drugs over the counter each year" (ExperienceLife.com/EXPERIENCE LIFE/). Prescription and over the counter drugs have become a way of life, for many people.

There are a few simple things that people can do to help themselves to become healthy again, and not over indulge in medications. Such as studying the Word of God and meditation of it; Worshipping God; eating well-balanced meals; drinking plenty of water; exercising, and getting the proper sleep. Most health issues can be corrected by just doing these simple things. God designed it that way in the beginning. What should happen when people go the doctor is to get their results and take them to the Lord in Prayer. When people pray, learn to trust God, and believe in that which He has promised, life situations will begin to change. When in doubt, God will give you the answer that you need if you seek His face. God is a healer, but people must believe and have faith in God that He is who He says He is.

CHAPTER ONE: HEALTH

I understand why some doctors do what they do concerning people's health. Medications are a remedy for a quick fix, but not a cure for the disease. If medicine was a cure, there would be no need to continue taking it. By definition, "cure is to treat illness successfully: to bring an end to an illness, disorder, or injury by medical treatment" (Webster Dictionary). Some doctors are afraid to give people other options for fear that they will not follow through and do what they need to do in order to get well. People in general; want to take the easy way out. They would rather take pills than to change their life styles. What they fail to consider is that most medications have some type of side effect. People take it for one health issue and end up with several other issues that stems from that one medication. I feel that people should be educated about the medication before it is taken. People should be told about the many side effects. They have options whether to take certain medications or not to take them. They just need to exercise these options.

Personally, I hate taking any type of medication whether it is a pill or liquid. I prefer to eat lot of fruits and vegetables instead of medication. I have a really big problem swallowing pills. Now, I believe it is God's way of letting me know that I do not need to put pills in my body which is the temple of the Lord. I do not want to contaminate my temple with any type of drug, therefore, I must be careful of the things that I put in God's Temple. God will destroy anyone who misuses His Temple. I learned to trust God with my health, and all of my other issues. God has the perfect healthcare plan---why not take advantage of this free gift?

It has been an eye-opener for me to see how people's lives can be turned upside down and inside out, just from taking prescription and nonprescription medications. God just wants us to trust Him with everything and stop trying to figure it out ourselves. Allow God to lead and guide you, and eliminate many of the health issues that you face each day. Poor health is not just an issue for adults, but children also have the same health concerns due largely to poor diet and unhealthy eating habits. It is important to get back to the basic; how God set it up in the beginning. The Scripture says, "And God said, Behold, I have given you every herb bearing tree, which is upon the face of all the earth, and every tree, in the which is the fruit of a tree yielding seed; to you it shall be for meat" (Genesis 1:2). This is God's perfect plan.

> Jorge Cruise explains, "Unhealthy diet—High dietary intakes of saturated fat, trans-fats and salt, and low intake of fruits and vegetables and fish are linked to cardiovascular risk, although whether all these associations are causal is disputed. The World Health organization attributes approximately 1.7 million deaths world-wide to low fruit and vegetable consumption. The amount of dietary consumed is also an important determinant of blood pressure level and overall cardiovascular risk. Frequent consumption of high-energy foods,

such as processed foods that are high in fats and sugars promote obesity and may increase cardiovascular risk".

(en.wikipedia.org/wiki/Jorge-Cruise 2010)

Some of the common health issues that men, women, and children are facing each day of their lives are related to diet and eating habits. They are as follow: Blood Pressure, Diabetes, Stroke, Heart Disease, Kidney Disease, Gout, and Cholesterol, to name a few. Women face issue such as Hot Flashes and Night Sweats. All of these issues can be corrected just by taking care of our bodies, changing our eating habits, and learning to balance life so that we don't get all stressed out. Jorge Cruise talks about the "hidden sugar" in food. According to his article, "Cruise therefore stresses the importance of reading labels for those "hidden sugar" which alleges also contributing to heart disease, cancer, and type II diabetes" (www.jorgecruise.com).

All of these things are important for healthy living, and long life. According to the Word of God, *"Beloved I wish above all things that thou may prosper and be in health, even as thy soul prospers"* (3 John 1:2). God wants us to live a bountiful and prosperous life. He wants us to do well and have good health. God wants His people to be healed. This is a promise from the Lord, who is a covenant keeper. We can begin to take control of our health issues by taking control of our souls (thoughts, will, and emotions...)

I write this book with one goal in mind: to help the people of God to become health conscience enough to change their lifestyles and begin to live their lives, abundantly, with dominion and power as God promised in His Word. The study of God's Word is so important if we are to know what He says about living. He does have an interest in our lives, if we allow him to, because He cares about what happens to each of us. My desire is to see the younger generation gain knowledge so they will not suffer as the older generation has suffered. It is not too late for

---

any generation to adapt, to change and want to live a healthy, prosperous life. I know how hard it is especially for my seasoned people to adapt to changes. Once your mind is made up, it is much easier to come up with all types of reasons why their situations cannot change or why they cannot do better. When people get older, making excuses seem to be the solution to the problem. Instead of putting the blame where it lies, God's people will blame everything on age, which is so far from the truth. Health issues arise generally because people have not taken proper care of themselves, over a lifetime. I don't blame them for their conditions, because most of us just didn't know any better.

The time has come whereas we should educate ourselves. Growing up on home remedies, I understand how much everything has changed. My grandmother used home remedies for our medical needs. There were no doctor visits or prescription drugs, except for emergency incidents. My grandmother had wisdom and motherly love, which came from God. They have yet to make the connection through the Word of God and that everything was provided for God's people back on Calvary by our Lord and Savior, Jesus Christ. I realize that some people will never make the connection that every good and perfect thing is tied to the Word of God.

People have been conditioned by society to expect certain things to happen to them when they reach a certain age. For instance, it's the norm for older people to believe that aches and pains, stiff joints, weak knees, and swelling of feet are just part of getting old. Also, they are known for consuming so much prescription drugs. By living according to God's Word and taking control of our lives, we can become a drug free society and I don't mean street drugs. According to a news report, August 16, 2013 over 16,000 people in America alone, died from drugs in 2012. I am speaking of prescription drugs, which is the number one killer in America, according to Dr. Gipson, who spoke at the Seasoned Olive's Conference, of The New Olivet Baptist Church, Memphis, TN. The causes stem from a combination of things, such as overdoses, wrong drugs prescribed, and taken incorrectly. As one doctor explains, "Researchers have discovered that many of the drugs that are imported from other countries are counterfeited, and are not good for Human consumption" (www.droz.com). It would be in your best interest to research all drugs.

Since I started writing this book, I have begun to hear more doctors speak out against prescription drugs and the harm caused by some drugs. Also, many pharmaceutical companies now take responsibility by pointing out major side effects that drugs may cause when they are consumed. The side effects of prescription drugs can cause other health problems. For example, BOTOX is a prescription drug that is injected into muscles and used to treat neurologic disease. We run the risk of becoming walking drug stores, bamboozled into thinking drug prescription is the only answer. The fact is, that in most cases, prescription drugs add to your health problems.

A magazine article from Allergan Pharmaceuticals explain, "Side effects of BOTOX include: dry mouth, tiredness, headache, neck pain, double vision, blurred vision, decreased eyesight, drooping eyelids, swelling of your eyelids, and dry eyes" www.allergan.com (Good Housekeeping Pg. 64, May 2014). I often wonder why anyone would consume medication that could do more harm than good to their health.

An NBC News Reporter recently stated, "Senior citizens' drug addiction is on the rise primarily from prescription drugs". Elderly people have become addicted to medication. Medication can be viewed as the pharmaceutical prison system. If you get caught up in the system, your resistance can be damaged, and you may be scared for the rest of your life. The more medication you put into your system, the more your body will crave it increasing the chance you will become hooked and "need" it for the rest of your life. As a society, we are led to believe that taking medicine is the only way that we will survive. Very few doctors are promoting natural, non-substance based healing for the body. The Scripture says, *"And the fruit thereof shall be for meat, and the leaf thereof for medicine"* (Ezekiel 47:12). God's Word has not changed; the same instructions apply to us today.

We are now living in a time where people are concerned with life, the economy and the state of the world; a serious society is careful about their bodies. People should realize they can't continue to consume any and everything. Sometimes, it's good to take a moment to think about the way things are. Pay attention and see the changing of time before our eyes. For example, child bearing has taken on a different meaning, with vastly different results. During my child bearing days, I was never sick, except for a few bouts of morning sickness every now and then. I was able to maintain my household duties, and I worked in my yard. I took care of a beautiful flower garden and a vegetable garden. I saw these chores as good exercise, a way to ensure a healthy pregnancy. The majority of women who become pregnant today are ill their entire pregnancy, have low energy levels before and after childbirth.

I spoke with a younger woman a few months ago, who was placed on bed rest for nine months. She shared with me she was not able to do anything for herself, and that someone had to care for her. My question is why such a big difference? What caused the difference? My next question is, why are there so many unhealthy babies being born today? During my child bearing days, these situations were rare. Of course, my thoughts are, the food that the mothers are consuming, not wearing proper clothing, and the medication they take, are contributors to this change. This is just one example; however, there are many examples of a decline in our health, particularly, women's health due to food choices. There was a time when people were more concerned about what they were going to eat than what medicine they were going to take. I am just old enough to see how so many things have changed, but were these changes better for you? Some changes have done more harm than good.

My goal is to increase your awareness and knowledge of food choices, so you may determine the changes needed in your food type. Below you will find a list of healthy food choices, to help you make the change.

FOOD CHOICES

Vegetables	Fruits	Nuts	Herbs
Asparagus	Apples	Acorns	Chia Seeds
Beans	Apricots	Almonds	Flaxseeds
Beets	Avocado	Cashews	Grape Seeds
Broccoli	Bananas	Brazils	Hemp Seeds
Brussels Sprouts	Blackberries	Peanuts	Pumpkin Seeds
Cabbage	Blueberries	Pecans	Sesame Seeds
Carrots	Cantaloupe	Pistachios	Sunflower Seeds
Cauliflower	Cherries	Walnuts	
Celery	Grapes		
Corn	Grapefruit		
Eggplant	Honeydew		
Garlic	Kiwifruit		
Greens	Lemons		
String Beans	Limes		
Kale	Mangoes		
Mushrooms	Oranges		
Okra	Peaches		
Onions	Pears		
Peas	Pineapple		
Spinach	Plums		
Squash	Raspberries		
	Strawberries		
	Tangerines		
	Watermelon		

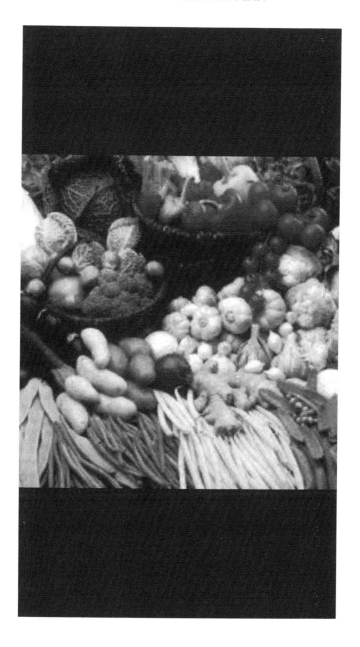

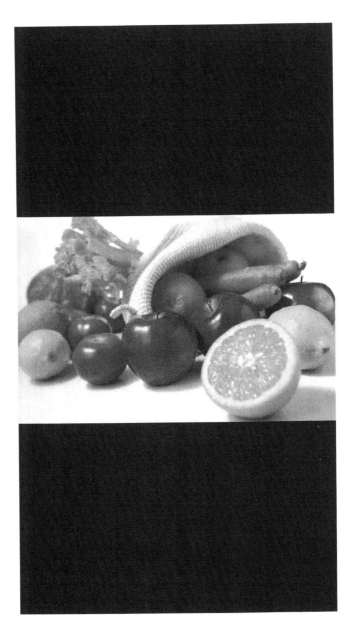

The big change is linked to the way food we are now consuming is being grown; which is very quickly. The normal growth of seed time and harvest is being altered to make vegetables and fruits grow faster. I was reared on a farm where my grandmother was a shared cropper; we grew our own food. We went through the normal seed, plant, and harvest process. In early spring, the soil was tilled for planting, and the seeds were planted. In late spring, and early summer, we would begin to gather food from our garden to eat. In late summer, and early fall, we would begin to gather vegetables and fruits for canning to carry us through the winter months. It was a lengthy process that included gathering the vegetables or fruits, shelling the beans or peas, shucking the corn, peeling the fruits, and washing everything, including the jars, so the food could be canned. My grandmother purchased a deep freezer when I was eleven, and we began to freeze much of our food, instead of canning. During the fall, we would gather nuts (pecans, peanuts, hickory nuts, and walnuts) to eat during the winter months. We raised our own hogs, cows, goats, chickens, geese, ducks, and turkeys. We also owned horses and mules.

As you can see, we bought very little food from the grocery store. We bought such food items as flour, meal, rice, grits, pasta, cereals, flavor, sugar, and syrup. Occasionally, she would buy meat and lard during the summer months. My grandmother made the buck of the lard from the fat of the hogs. Our sausage, smoke sausage, ham, and bacon from the hogs we raised, which were all natural without additives. Our milk and butter came from the cows, and our eggs came from our chickens. She also made our jelly from grapes and muscadines. Economically, this was the way we survived. My grandmother had very little money to spend for food. What money she had, was used for other necessities such as, utilities, burial insurance, kerosene oil, and school supplies.

Basically, we grew most of the foods we ate, naturally

grown without chemicals. Manure from the cows was used as a fertilizer for our garden. We used Mother Nature's products which consisted of fresh vegetables, fruits, and nuts for our medication. The home remedies were used occasionally to keep our bodies well such as, Castor Oil for colds, Father John's for colds and flu, 366 for colds, floured water for diarrhea, hog hoof tea for whooping cough, mullein leaves for swelling, beef (fat) for chest colds, Black Draught and Epsom Salt for laxative.

A few people still plant gardens and raise their own meat, but the majority people depend on grocery stores and farmer's markets for their food supplies, including people in rural areas. Farming is past history; more people are working in office and factory jobs. They have no time for planting gardens or raising anything. The lard I mentioned above, I will never use to prepare food these days. It contains trans-fat which is bad for our bodies. It has been associated with heart diseases and obesity. When you obtain knowledge that a food item is not healthy for you, you must be willing to make the change in order to have a well-body. Don't continue to use it and take risks. Take it off of the "good" list and replace it with something better! This is a Biblical Principle in action, when we know better, we must do better.

It makes me so sad when I see people continue to use products they know are not good for them. For instance, most medications we take have known side effects, but we continue to take them anyway because we hope the good will out way the bad. As if to say, "I don't care about the consequences; I just want a quick fix." After we have messed up our bodies with medications, we ask God to fix the problem, make us whole again. Yet, God is saying I was there all the time, but you chose to seek help from other sources first. Throughout our lives making God the last resort can be a sign of distrust. In reality, He should be the first source that we seek for help and guidance. Anything else, including medicine should be secondary.

Pastor Joseph Prince says, "When you receive God's Word as truth, you will see your healing and deliverance from every evil condition sent to destroy you" (www.josephprince.org/.../receiving-healing-with-faith-and-patience)! God knows everything that is to be known about our lives. If you seek God's help and guidance first, He will connect you to the right source. Sometimes your human side will make you believe that there are some things that you shouldn't bother to take to God. Any foolishness, no, you shouldn't bother Him, but anything concerning your health, you should seek Him first.

Beware! Over-the-counter pain relievers and vitamin supplements are bad news, including aspirins. For many years, people have been made to believe that an aspirin a day would prevent blood clots. Now, researchers have discovered it was all a myth. According to a magazine article written by Kristin Ohlson, "Because they've been told over and over to take low doses of aspirin to protect their hearts, most people are surprised to hear that aspirin pose cardiac risks" (Experience Life.com/pg. 64 June 2014). Unless you have suffered a heart attack or heart problems, you should not be taken any aspirin. You should rely upon the Holy Spirit for guidance, because he will not lead you wrong. If you worship, pray, believe, trust, and act on God's Word, it will keep you on the right path.

I never shall forget a few years ago, I was driving and listening to the radio, there was a promotion going on, for the month of February, around Valentine's Day. The radio announcer said, "You can receive a free heart test and also receive a free gift by registering," and the announcer went on to give the information on how to register. I thought to myself, maybe I should register to have the heart test done. The Holy Spirit spoke to me, "Don't waste those people's time because there is nothing wrong with your heart." Immediately, that idea vanished from my thoughts. That's why I rely upon the Holy Spirit to lead and direct me, because He knows all there is to know about me (and you).

If you trust Him, He will not allow you to be deceived by anyone. He will keep you alert of the perpetrators.

Many elderly people spend so much money buying medications each month, so much so, that, after buying their medications, they barely have enough money left to take care of other necessities. The cost of medical care goes up each year, even though most of them have Medicare, which only covers part of the out of pocket cost for their medical expenses. They are very loyal to the medical advice that says they need the pills in order to survive. I am here to say, the pills are not the solution, but they substitute for the answer that can fix the problem.

I have spoken with people who take four pills for high blood pressure daily, and their blood pressure is still high. This should let you know that something is very wrong. The listed side effects from the pills probably have caused even more health problems for the person. For example, people who are taking medication for high blood pressure will more likely end up taking medication for diabetes, as a known correlation exists between untreated high blood pressure and diabetes. Most of the time, doctors don't know which medications will work and may try a number of alternatives and hope the medication prescribed will solve the problem and not create new medical issues. Notice, I didn't say praying that the medication will work, because many health professional do not acknowledge the concept of the power of prayer. Regardless of where or how you receive medical advice, it is important that you do some research before you start, or continue taking prescription drugs after seeing side effects. You need to find out the type of side effect it has before you start taking any medication. Once certain medications get in your system, they can possibly become habit forming, and the body will begin to crave it, and cause harm.

There have been several occasions where my doctor prescribed medication and I refused to take it. The first time, my cholesterol was high and I was given medication to take, well I didn't take any of that medication. I did my own research to determine natural remedies and steps I could take, on my own. I confided in my sister about my high cholesterol. She shared that oatmeal lowed her cholesterol over time. I went to the store and I bought old-fashion oatmeal which worked for me. I began to eat oatmeal every day, with cinnamon and honey, lowed my cholesterol over time. Steel-cut, all natural oatmeal is preferred. December 31, 2012 glucose (sugar) was found in my urine. Again, I refused to take the medication. This was on New Year's Eve. I went to the altar to lay prostrate before the LORD (The Eternally Self Existent One, Who Keeps His Covenant Promises to His Covenant People) and the Holy Spirit began to minister to me. Normally, you have sugar in your urine because you have been eating sweets. It was after the Christmas Holiday and I had eaten quite a bit of the sweet stuff. Immediately, I stopped eating sweets, and about a month later, I had my glucose checked again. It was eighty-eight, which is considered fine. I believe: had I taken the medication, I would have developed diabetes. I am so grateful to God for His wisdom and guidance. It is always wise to be aware of what you are putting in your body, because you might be doing more harm than good.

Recently I came across several quotations from an expert that sums up his experience with blood sugar: "Anything under 100 is considered fine, but even with my healthy diet and all my intensive fitness training, my levels were still in the 90's, which felt a little too close for comfort."

"I'd already cut out most processed sugar, so after doing some research, I started experimenting with removing flour and processed grains, too."

"Very quickly, my fasting blood sugar dropped to the mid-80s. I felt better, and my athletic training improved. Eating this way, I also dropped about 20 lbs. in 90 days, getting down to my leanest racing weight yet" according to

Bahram Akradi, who is the founder and CEO of Life Time Fitness. I am so grateful to have researched and found resources to support my belief.

In August, 2004, my mother, who was sixty-nine went to the hospital for about two weeks. The doctor was treating her for a respiratory infection. She had diabetes and high blood pressure. After she came home from the hospital, I went home to Mississippi to spend some time with her and to take care of her for a few days. I was looking forward to having a great time with my mother. I had big plans for the days we were going to spend together. On my way there, that Thursday evening, I stopped at the store to purchase food so I could cook a big meal. I got up very early the next morning to start my day. I made breakfast so my mother could eat and take her medications after she got up. After breakfast, I began to clean and I cooked the rest of the food. I cooked enough food to last for quite a while, because I didn't want her to worry about cooking anything after I left. Also, this would give her more time to recuperate before returning to her daily chores. I wanted to make everything comfortable for her, and ease some of her burden, while I was there. She never got a chance to enjoy any of it. I didn't know how ill my mother really was at that time.

After I finished cooking, I fixed her plate. She tried to eat, but she was only able to eat a very small amount. Little did I know; my mother was very sick! By her bed was a small table where she kept all of her medications. On that table were thirteen different medications and the hospital sent one by carrier that day which made fourteen. I asked my mother if she thought she should be taking all of that medication, and she said, "Yes, that's what my doctor told me to take." She never questioned the doctor about the many medications; she just took what her doctor prescribed. I thought to myself, why so many medications. As I thought about it later on, there was no way she could have kept all of the medicines and instructions straight in

20

her head. It was too much stuff for any one person to take at one time. Even though she had the spiritual authority, (a believer) she never consulted with God concerning her medication. It was as if she thought God could not be reached. Yet, she never asked her doctor any questions about her medication, because she trusted him to make the right decision about her health.

About six o'clock that Friday evening, mother became very ill and I had to call the ambulance to rush her to the emergency room. I am so glad God allowed me to be there when she became ill. I took all her medications to the hospital and the medical person that admitted my mother could not tell me what conditions some of those medications were ever prescribed to treat. After hours of waiting in the emergency room, the doctor finally came in to check her out. She was moved to a room about 3:00 A.M., in the morning. I went back to her home and put the food in containers to be frozen and to pick-up some items for her. I had to get my belongings so I could return home to Memphis that evening. She stayed there for a few days for more testing, but the doctors could not find what was actually wrong with her. I noticed that my mother appeared to have gained a lot of weight. I found out later that it was fluid build-up in her body. She kept saying to me, "I have got to lose this weight." The doctor finally, recommended she come to Memphis for further testing.

The doctors in Memphis ran more tests on her, and discovered that her heart was in bad condition. She had arterial blockages that required immediate surgery. On August 13, 2004, she had surgery and she came through the surgery fine. One week later, and one day before her 70th birthday, she became very ill, and they discovered that she had blood clots around her heart, which required them to perform a second surgery. I rushed to the hospital where I continued to pray to God for my mother to recover from surgery. Father, in the name of Jesus, I come before you; lifting up my mother, who is going through surgery. I know you are with my mother; guiding the surgeon's hands. Heavenly Father, continue to grant your healing power Amen. I found out later she stopped breathing twice during surgery, but she was revived. I prayed for my mother, and God answered my prayer.

I know God would have given her the right answer, had she only asked Him. Trust in God and not man, because man will deceive us. When it comes to my health, I have learned to trust God to help me make the right decision. Since He knows everything about me, why not consult a reliable source when we need an answer? We must remember if it's in His Will, God will fix it. That's why we must check with God first.

Over the next few months, she improved some, but never fully recovered. She was released from the hospital in October and sent to Hartland Rehabilitation Center, 6060 Walnut Grove Memphis, TN, for treatment. She appeared to be getting better, but on November 20, 2004, she had another episode, was rushed back to the hospital and put on a ventilator until she was able to breathe on her own. There was very little improvement after this ordeal. On December 13, 2004, I celebrated my birthday with my family. The next day, I got a call from the hospital that it was not looking good for her. My family and I went to the hospital and prayed. She appeared to be some better. After we left the hospital, took my brother to the bus station, I went home. About two hours later, I received a call from the hospital saying that we needed to return to the hospital because my mother's condition had gotten worse. When we arrived at the hospital, on December 15, 2004 my mother had passed. I called my brother who was on the bus going home to share with him that mother had passed. This was two days after my birthday.

As I am writing, I am reminded of the pain and suffering that she had gone through during her illness. I don't want to go through this type of suffering, nor do I want anyone else to suffer. After my mother's death, I began to look at health from a different perspective. After my mother's ordeal with her health issues, the Holy Spirit began to show me some things that were going on in the world around me. It made me realize that something was not right. I have come to realize that much of our suffering is our own fault when it comes to our health, because we take so many things for granted. We must take the initial step when it comes to our health, to ensure we are doing all that we can do to maintain good health, for long life.

My mother's health situation was an eye opener for me. It also made me realize how little I knew about my mother's health condition. I knew she had diabetes, high blood pressure, and occasionally she was treated for respiratory problems. I had no idea that my mother had heart problems until she came to Memphis. She arrived in Memphis that Tuesday afternoon, and the doctor began testing her that Wednesday morning. When the results came back, it was discovered that she had ninety percent heart blockage. The doctor at the hospital advised that she needed immediate surgery in order to survive. She went to surgery that Thursday. The lesson I learned from that ordeal was that we need to check on our parents and the elderly in our communities and pay close attention to their health issues. I know sometimes parents can be very secretive about what is really going on in their lives, fearing they will place a burden on us. But, any caring child or children would want to know what is going on with their parents. We should care about the well-being of our parents. Even if they didn't do everything that we thought that they should have done, we should want the best of care for them.

Heart diseases or heart problems have been the major cause of death on the maternal side of my family for generations. I remembered grandmother's uncle had a heart attack and died from it, and my maternal grandmother died from a massive heart attack. I am paying close attention to my family's health history so those things do not happen to me. That's why I pay attention to the foods that I consume. I am going to do everything in my power to make sure this generational cycle does not repeat itself. God has given me power to control some things in my life---I must have enough will power to be in charge over those things that will cause me problems later on in life. I am not going to let the enemy destroy my health or my life. I am going to use the weapon that God has given me, which is His Word, to destroy Satan and all the demons that are on assignment for him. I have been equipped by God to do battle against Satan, through the Word of God.

When I study the Word of God, I become aware of the enemy's tricks and the Holy Spirit keeps me abreast of everything the enemy tries pull over on me. I know it is Satan who wants to harm me, and not God. That's why it pays to stay in the Will of God. His Will keeps me safe and protects me from all dangers. As long as I am in the Will of God, I am well covered and there is nothing for me to be concerned about. God keeps a close watch over me, and no harm will come upon me. The Scripture says, *"No weapon that is formed against thee shall prosper; and every tongue that shall rise against thee in judgment thou shalt condemn. This is the heritage of the servants of the LORD, and their righteousness is of me, says the LORD"* (Isaiah 54:17). They will form, but they cannot hurt me.

We should never lose our focus, because God has a purpose and a plan for each of us. He determined from the beginning how our lives would be designed, and He designed it just for us. He tells us in His word, how we should live and what we should do and what we should not do, in order to live holy. We should not fall for the Devil's tricks, which make us believe that because someone in our family had certain diseases, we are going to have the same diseases. The Scripture says, *"In those days they shall say no more, the fathers have eaten a sour grape, and the children's teeth are set on edge"* (Jeremiah 31:29 KJV). I have already decreed and declared to Satan that I will not have the diseases of my mother, grandmother, and uncle.

God has given us the power to determine our own destiny, by speaking life into existence. We must be careful of the things that we speak, whether they are positive or negative. I have heard people say my grandmother, mother, and father had it, it runs in the family, so it must be hereditary. Well, it does not matter who had that disease in your family. You do not have to claim any disease that ran in the family. God declared, *"If thou will diligently hearken to the voice of the LORD thy God, and will do that which is right in His sight, and give ear to His commandments, and keep all of His statutes, I will put none of these diseases upon thee, which I have brought upon the Egyptians: for I am the LORD that heals thee"* (Exodus 15:26). The Egyptians were plagued with leprosy because of their disobedience against God's laws. God gives instructions through His Word how we can avoid sicknesses and diseases. We do not want to be stiff-necked and hard hearted when it comes to obeying the word of God. This is LORD, JEHOVAH God, the One who keeps His covenant promises to His covenant people. Here, God was speaking to the Israelites which also apply to us today. God is saying to us to today if you will listen to my voice, through my Word, and act accordingly, you are already healed.

There is nothing under the sun that cannot be changed or corrected according to God's Word. You can begin to change some things by speaking them into existence. The Scripture says, *"Death and life are in the power of the tongue: and they that love it shall eat the fruit thereof"* (Proverbs 18:21). If you are in good standing with God, you can begin to use your tongue to speak life and not death: to speak healing and not sickness. There is power in the tongue and we must make sure this power is used correctly, because if used incorrectly, it could be used to work against us. This does not mean that you are dotting all the I's and crossing all of the T's, but you should be living a God kind of life to the best of your ability, and please God. When we fall short in certain areas of our lives, we must repent to God who is just to forgive us of our sins. We want to always speak life and not death. We can have life through our Lord and Savior Jesus Christ, and have it more abundantly. We must remember what God said back then, still holds true for today's society.

We can change things just by verbally speaking them. Romans 4:17 states, *"And call those things which be not as though they were."* The Scripture says to speak those things into existence as though they were already happening; therefore, they shall come to past. It's a mind thing which I will address later on in the book. People must be careful about the things that they allow to enter their mind. I keep a positive mind and outlook of life. God has never allowed me to just settle for anything, concerning my body. Even when I did not fully understand this principle, I am so grateful to Him for keeping me. I have been blessed to know that there is a better way of _doing_ things, and so can you. It does not matter how we have always done things in the past. We should have an open mind when it comes to doing things in a more excellent way. That's why I want to help God's people make the transition from bad health to good health, through the Word of God.

CHAPTER TWO: WHY IS OUR HEALTH IMPORTANT TO GOD?

God wants us healthy to be able to meet our spiritual obligations. If we are ill, we cannot carry out God's will and do His work effectively. We must be able to do God's Kingdom work here on earth. God uses His people to build His Kingdom. We must live healthy lives in order to stay physically fit for the Kingdom of God. Some people have it twisted, because they think that retirement means to become a sitter and do nothing. Well not so; God does not have a retirement plan for anyone. We must continue to move until He says our labor is finished. We must keep in mind that we were created to be His servants, and He does not need any spectators who are doing nothing at all. We must continue to work and focus on good health in order to be effective servants, not **lazy, obese, unhealthy Christians**.

God began to deal with me a few years ago concerning the importance of good health. This was before I was called into the ministry. He began to make me become more and more concerned with other people's health issues. I began to speak to some people about their health issues as the Holy Spirit gave me knowledge. I knew my task would not be an easy one, because when people are set in their ways, they do not want to be corrected. Especially, those who are addicted to food, and when they feel you are trying to tell them what they should or should not eat. For it is such a personal choice, that people will begin to avoid you, and become very defensive when it comes to talking about food. They don't want to be told anything about the food they are consuming. Even today, as I write this book, I know some will get it and others will not. I know that I must keep doing what thus says the Lord.

Good health is my passion, and I must continue this journey, because I am on a mission for God, my Lord and Savior, Jesus Christ. My mission is to save God's people from destruction caused by health issues that have become a major problem in our society. I thank God for those people who believe in the Word of God and know that they can be set free through faith and trusting in God's Word. They should get to know God through His word. The Scripture says, *"Study to show yourself approved unto God, a workman that need not be ashamed, rightly dividing the word of truth"* (II Timothy 2:15). If God said it, believe me, it's very important that we do so. God wants us to study, to equip ourselves for warfare. Without the Word of God, we are as empty vessels, and cannot do battle against Satan. God's Word is our weapon against Satan and the sin of the world. By studying God's Word, we learn how to protect ourselves from the tricks of the enemy. His mission is to destroy God's people by any means necessary. He is doing a good job through the food that we are consuming. Satan uses things against us that we would never think of as a weapon to harm us, because he knows that we are easy prey when it comes to our desires.

Our good health plays a major role in each of our lives. When you are in good health, you are rich and you are able to do so many more positive things, such as focusing, creating, and looking for a better future each day that God allows you to see. You don't allow yourself to get caught up in what you haven't done, what you don't have in the present, but what you could have in the future. Good health keeps you full of energy and excitement which makes you want to do exciting things. Every day that God wakes you up, you should find something to be grateful and excited about. When you focus on excitement, there is no room for worry or fear over anything, and you can be content with your life. Excitement can lead to longevity which means that God keeps on adding years to your life. When you are excited about life, you will make sure to do the things that keep you healthy. You will find ways to stay healthy and maintain a healthy life-style. When you rely upon God for strength, He will help you give up those things that are not healthy; this means anything with the potential to destroy your body. Those foods that are not healthy, you will begin to eat them in moderation or give up over time.

I will list foods that we should incorporate in our daily diet. Our bodies need 3 to 5 servings of green leafy vegetables daily such as turnip, mustard, collard, rape, kale, spinach, and cabbage. Also, one pound of live food should be eaten daily, which is any combination of raw vegetables. 2 to 3 servings of fruits of your choice should be eaten daily, which should equal to one pound. 2 to 3 servings of nuts should be eaten daily (one ounce each) of any combination. Nuts are a good healthy snack between meals. 2 to 3 serving of meat (three ounces each) can be eaten daily. Again, there is no healing from meat; your healing comes from vegetables, fruits, grain, and nuts. 2 to 3 servings of bread (100% whole grain wheat) can be eaten daily. Be careful, when selecting bread, because 100% whole wheat is not the same as 100% whole grain wheat. These are your healthier choices of foods. Sweets should be eaten sparingly (moderation), and with a complete meal.

CHAPTER THREE:
BEING USED BY GOD

I am only a vessel being used by God to deliver His message to His people. Those that will receive God's knowledge will reap the benefit of God's promises. David says, *"Bless the LORD, O my soul, and forget not all His benefits: Who forgives all thine iniquities; who heals all thy diseases"* (Psalm 103:2-3). Here, David praises God for His mighty acts and the list goes on about the things that God does for his people. Mastering good health is not a hard thing to do, but we must discipline ourselves accordingly. Most importantly, we must rely upon the Holy Spirit who gives self-control and temperance in all things. There are many ways to practice self-control. For example, when your clothes begin to feel tighter, don't go out and buy a larger size. You should cut back on your food portions, watch what you eat, and exercise more. This does not mean that you have to stop eating, but you should make some minor changes in your diet and routine.

You must begin to develop a healthy eating pattern for your body. So many people don't want to discipline themselves so, instead of changing their eating habits, they take pills. Pills are a quick fix, but they cannot correct the initial problem. They are not a cure for the body. If the pills could cure the body, there would be no need to continue taking them. Many health issues are corrected just by changing your lifestyle. While it may seem hard to do, it is not impossible. Instead of giving up, make up your mind that you are going to live a healthy lifestyle. We must learn how to eat to live and not live just to eat.

It appears that it is difficult for people to understand that some foods are not as healthy as they once were, because of how they are grown and the chemicals that are used. It is important to closely screen what we eat. There are so many fake foods on the market today which appear to be at the top of the line, and they taste good, but they are not good for you. They have many additives, and fewer nutrients, which are not good for our bodies. Since I am being used by God in this area, it is often very difficult to warn people about some of the foods they are consuming. Sometimes they become very agitated and defensive when I tell them about some of the foods that are not good for them. I have learned people do not want to be told what to eat and what not to eat.

There are people who would rather consume pills just to be able to eat whatever they want, whether good or bad. I have heard the statement, "When I take my high blood pressure pill, I can eat whatever I want." At that point, you are treating your body like a garbage dump, putting in all kinds of trash. People are often so obsessed with food that before they can finish breakfast, they are already planning lunch and all the in-between meals. They don't spend much time thinking about anything else, especially not God's plan for their lives. I see so many people in today's society who are not concerned at all about their health. They just want to be able to consume as much food as possible, without anyone pointing out to them what is wrong. They don't realize that there are foods that are good for the body and other foods that are harmful to the body. I have learned when it comes to food people do not make good judgment. It goes back to our mind-set, expressing our free will, to obtain that which is good. What we want appears to have more value than what we need. We must condition our minds to work with the needs of our bodies, and not against them. We should use our mind to control our body and not our mouth.

Every thought and every deed begins with the mind, whether it's good or bad. Focus on the positive things and not the negative things of life; it is very important and a key to happiness. If you allow the Holy Spirit to control your mind, you can accomplish your goals and have the desires of your heart. The Scripture says, *"I can do all things through Christ that strengthen me"* (Philippians 4:13). When you condition your mind, all things are possible. The mind is where it all begins; therefore, the mind must be programmed with sound information from the Word of God. We must take control of our mind and not allow the enemy's control.

Satan will use our mind to play all types of tricks on us. For example, he will make you believe that you are sick and you will never be healed. You are poor and you will never be rich. You are a failure and you will never be successful. You are a loser and you will never be a winner. We can reverse and destroy every one of Satan's trick with the Word of God. For example, we can use I AM factors, "I am the head and not tail; I am above and not beneath; I am a lender and not a borrower." Even though Satan won't just give up, we can block his view into our life with the Word of God. The Scripture says, *"Submit yourselves therefore to God. Resist the devil, and he will flee from you. Draw nigh to God and He will draw nigh to you"* (James 4:7-8). We must not allow our minds to get tangled up in Satan's mess. If he gets your mind, he will control your life. He will block every blessing that God has for you. When he conquers your mind, he makes you think that you don't need God. We must remember that God wants what is best for us and we should want the best for our selves.

God created everything we needed in the beginning. He put in place a perfect plan and purpose for our lives until man messed up; then everything changed. When Adam and Eve were in the Garden of Eden, God had their destiny already planned. They were to be obedient and do according to the Word of God---which was to be "fruitful and multiply." Adam and Eve were to set the example for the human race. They allowed the enemy to distract them from God's divine plan, which caused them to get off track. The enemy is always trying to get us to disobey and distrust God. He makes everything look good, taste good, and feel good. I suspect that the fruit that Adam and Evil ate in the Garden had the same effect on them. Satan does not have any new tricks. He is using the same old tricks that he used on Eve in the Garden of Eden. Everything was great before he showed up. His job is to put wedges among God and His people which cause separation from God. He knows when we get distracted and we are separated from God, we are more easily persuaded by his tricks. That's why it is so important for us to guard our minds.

Satan hasn't just started playing this mind game. He has been playing mind games for a very long time. He started with Eve when he tricked her into eating the forbidden fruit, and she gave it to Adam to do likewise. At that point, Adam should have reminded Eve of the instructions that God had given to him, about the forbidden fruit. Then, he tried to blame Eve for his action, but God never gave Eve any instructions; He gave them to Adam. After Adam and Eve disobeyed God's command, they suffered the consequences for their actions. Being removed from the Garden of Eden was one of the consequences for their disobedience to God's command. It was ordered by God that Adam and Eve would never return to the Garden of Eden. As you can see, this consequence was for the rest of their lives.

We too will be held accountable for our own actions. When we are disobedient to the Word of God, we will pay the price and suffer the consequences that come with sin. Yes, God does forgive us of all of our sins, but the consequences can follow us for the rest of our lives. It is the sin that God erases and puts in the sea of forgetfulness, but not the consequences. You get to keep those, and they could last for life. Consequences are like thorns in the flesh, we learn to live with them, but are never rid of them. God does forgive us for every one of our sins, but the consequences remain our concern.

It appears that people don't give much thought to consequences, and seem to believe that when they are forgiven for their sin the debt is settled. If people gave more thought to their consequences, they would be more careful about some of their actions in life. Bad eating habits lead to bad health, which is the consequence of not eating right. I challenge you to make the change and see the result of a new body and life.

Bad eating habits cause us to have major health problems in life. There is a correct way to do anything. Believe me! I know that old habits are hard to break, but they can be broken through prayer and discipline. Some things we have done for so long until they seem like the right thing to do. For example, drinking liquid while you are eating is a bad habit. No one should eat and drink liquid at the same time. You should drink liquid before you eat or after you eat, but you should never drink liquid with food. Food is a solid, and is better digested and more nutritious for the body when consumed alone. I know that some people feel that food needs to be 'washed' down, but that is just an old wives tale that we have heard for a long time. Mixing solids and liquids together cause you to eat more. "Eating and drinking can cause you to eat more, because you wash the food out of the porch," according to Dr. Robert Wegner. Also, you have that bloated feeling making you uncomfortable, and it feels as if you are going to pop. Again, when you know better, you should do better. Drinking water before you eat is better than having a beverage while eating.

Water is natural without any additive, and filler as well as a purifier and is very good for the body. Another concept is that when you drink water before you eat, you will not eat as much which is very good for people who are trying to cut back. The body makeup is seventy percent water; that's why it is so important to consume the proper amount of water each day. I know water can be a big problem for some people, but there are things you can do to enhance your water such as lemon, lime, cucumber, strawberry, and other berries. Water is life and it will make the soul merry.

CHAPTER FOUR:
WHAT EXAMPLES ARE WE SETTING
FOR OUR CHILDREN?

We, as parents, are setting bad examples for our children, when we allow our children to develop bad eating habits. I have seen toddlers sitting at the table to eat, and they have a cup of soda larger than them. They will begin drinking the soda before eating their foods most times they will drink the soda and leave their food, which means they have gotten very little nutrition from their meal. If the parents threaten to remove the soda, they become upset. Guess who wins? The children do, because the parents do not want to deal with the upset child.

There are some things I never allowed my children to do, like drinking beverages while eating or going out-side to play in church or school clothing. They had to finish their food and then they could drink their beverages. My reason at the time for not allowing them to drink while eating was to make sure that they had a wholesome meal. I wanted to make sure they got nutrition from the food. I knew if I had allowed them to drink while eating, they would not have eaten their food. I never allowed them to play in church or school clothing for fear of them ruining their Sunday best or school best. Not once, did any of them ever ask why they could not have their beverages with their meal or why they had to change their clothing, because they knew the rules and they understood. I had no idea at the time this was the way we should eat. Although, it was the way I had been taught as a child. After I got grown, I tried a few times to eat and drink, but it never worked for me. I would get full and I could hardly finish my food. It made me miserable and I didn't like that feeling. So I stopped, now I drink before or after eating, but never with my food. I understand why we should not drink anything while we are eating our meal.

The next problem I see is that small children are given too much candy, which is bad for their teeth and it also causes them to become hyperactive, unruly and out of control. Then, the parents are wondering what is wrong with their children. They are on a sugar high from the candy. Sheila Mulrooney Eldred says, "A few years ago, researchers discovered that the artificial colors Yellow No 5 and Yellow No 6 promote Attention Deficit Disorder (ADD) in children. In fact, Norway and Sweden have already banned the use of these artificial colors, and in the rest of the EU, food containing these additives must be labeled with the phrase:" "May have an adverse effect on activity and attention in children" (Experience Life.com). We wonder why young people have so many health problems. Not to mention all the fast foods they are consuming.

Recent research study shows an increase in children who are affected by some type of behavior problems such as, ADHD (attention deficit hyperactivity disorder) and ADD (attention deficit disorder). Most of these children are prescribed medication for these symptoms which has not solved the problem. I have observed children who have been prescribed medication; they appear to be in a state of confusion.

Most children are eating some type of fast food every day and nobody knows for sure what is in the meat or the greasy fries. Children should not be eating this type of food every day; it should be eaten in moderation, like special occasions. Food Babe talks about how her parents immigrated to the United States from India. Her dad allowed her and her brother to fit into the American lifestyle. Her mother would prepare two meals---a meal for herself and their dad which was the Indian food from scratch---which she thought was gross. And for the children, she relied on processed foods: microwavable Salisbury steak, mozzarella sticks, chicken tenders and all that stuff from the frozen section. They were allowed to eat whatever they wanted, including McDonald's, Burger King and Wendy's. They wanted to fit in the world around them. VANI HARI (the Food Babe) says, "I was sick as a child. I never wanted to go to school. I always had a stomachache. I had eczema all over my body, Asthma and Allergies. I was in and out of the doctor's office all the time" (ExperienceLife.com). Her illness was linked to the food that she was consuming.

I have never seen so many obese children in the recent years of my life. Medical officials are still trying to determine whether or not there is link between youth obesity and fast foods consumption. Young mothers are so busy doing other things until they can't find time to cook or they can't cook. I realize that there are single parent homes where the mothers have to work, but those that can cook should find the time to cook a wholesome meal for their children as often as they can. They can cook enough to last for a few days so that the children are fed well. Children must be taught at an early age to eat healthy. If they are not taught to eat healthy, the fast foods become a way of life for them. Life must have balance and the parents should find ways to create balance. Our children are hurting because of the lack of cooking in the home. Some of our children don't know anything about vegetables and fruits, or how healthy they are for their bodies. All they see is a fast food meal; therefore, if it's not a hamburger, hot dog or fries, they will refuse to eat.

Education at an early age should include the importance of healthy eating. Children are being diagnosed with the same diseases as the adults such as high blood pressure, diabetes, heart diseases and cancer. When they grow up, they are statistically labelled for bad health issues, due to a life of bad eating habits. Most people are so caught up in life issues that they are losing the battle on their health. We as a people have got to get back to the basics. As mothers, we should assess the care we provide to our family. Let's use the example of the Proverbs 31 woman, who looked out for the well-being of her family. The Scripture says, *"She looked well to the ways of her household, and eat not the bread of idleness. Her children arise up, and call her blessed; her husband also, and he praised her"* (Proverbs 31:27-28). She spent her time wisely making sure that her family's needs were taken care of, and that her household was prosperous. We, as (wives/mothers), are obligated to do likewise by taking responsibility for our family's health.

Like the Proverbs 31 woman, I took very good care of my family. I realize that I represent a different generation. I made sure my family had a home cooked meal every day. I even made their hamburgers and fries, which they only ate on some Fridays and Saturdays. I made sure that they had a wholesome meal. I did not allow my children to choose the food they wanted to eat. I cooked, put it on their plates, and they ate what I cooked. They did not have a choice in the matter. They were kept neat, clean and hair combed. As I mentioned earlier, my children were not allowed to play in church or school clothing; therefore, they had three sets of clothing. They had a church set, school set and a play set. As a wife and a mother, I had the responsibility of taking care of my family that God had placed in my care. I am the caretaker and the overseer of my family; God designed it that way. There is no place in society for a lazy female then or now. As mothers, we should be the first teachers that our children see. We should teach them and bring them up according to God's Word.

Fathers also play a major role in their children lives. Fathers are the head of their family. They are providers for their family; God designed it that way. One of the biggest problems with our children today, is the absence of fathers in homes. Children are hurting from this ordeal; it affects their lives in many ways. Attention deficit hyperactivity disorder (ADHD) found in children's behavior, could be link to absent fathers. Children are happier when they see both parents getting along and working together. Fathers have that natural firmness, whereas, when they look or speak, they get respect from their children. For example, my children's father could speak, and from the sound of his voice tears began to roll down their cheeks. Whereas, when I spoke, no tears would fall, until I reached for the rod (paddle). The Scripture says, *"Train up a child the way he should go: and when he is old, he will not depart from it"* (Proverbs 22:6). As parents are responsible for molding and shaping our children's lives so that they can grow up to be dependable adults and make sound decisions, particularly about health and family.

Parenting must become a priority in the home. Many believe that a lack of parenting skills in the home has caused the children in today's society to go astray. Many parents are busy working and doing other things and they are missing out on the most important thing in their children lives, and that is parenting. Today children come home to be entertained by the TV, telephone or some type of electronic game that has little educational value. This type of influence can be dangerous for the minds of children which are not developed enough to determine the difference between what is real and what is make-believe. Parents and communities should guard our children from this type of influence. It can be extremely difficult for single parents to work, watch, and guard their children, but it can be done. Again, we must go back to the Word of God which teaches us how it should be done.

In today's society we seek experts, read their books and consult other avenues to find the answers on parenting. The Bible has the answer to everything that they need to know about parenting. God's Word is always true, and if we would govern ourselves accordingly, we could eliminate many of the problems that parents are facing today. While there are many good books out there, the Bible is the best and the most important book of all. It contains so much good information, and it gives detail instructions for parenting. The Scripture says, *"He that spare the rod hate his son: but he that love him chasten him betimes"* (Proverbs 13:24). The Bible is the only reliable source of knowledge and direction that we can count on to be true for our lives.

Loving parents will teach their children to obey authority, and when they become disobedient, they will discipline them in love. According to the Word of God, children should obey their parents while they are under their authority. The Scripture says, *"Children, obey your parents in the Lord: for this is right. Honor thy father and mother; which is the first commandment with promise; that it may be well with thee, and thy may live long on the earth"* (Ephesians 6:1-3). This same passage appears in the Old Testament as part of the Ten Commandments which is found in Exodus 20:12, and the only commandment that has a promise attached. We must teach our children the Ten Commandments so that they may begin to understand the instructions that God has given us to live by. Parents must teach their children to obey the Word of God.

There is much emphasis put on honor for thy father and thy mother. Another passage states, *"Honor thy father and thy mother, as the LORD thy God hath commanded thee; that thy days may be prolonged, and that it may go well with thee, in the land which the LORD thy God giveth thee"* (Deuteronomy 5:16). According to the Word of God, disobedient children days will be shortened on earth. When I look at today's society and the young people who are being killed every day, I am beginning to wonder if there is a connection to this passage. I just believe everything the Word of God says, and believe in the importance of teaching children the Word of God at an early age. Parents must set the foundation for our children's lives, with the expectation of good health and long life.

There should be rules and guidelines put in place for children to follow. Children should have chores around the house. They should be taught to help maintain their home and to pick up after themselves. Children need to have some type of responsibilities. They need a set time for going to bed each night and their TV turned off at that time. Children who spend a lot of time watching TV, which decreased the time spent on the more positive things of life. Research shows a need for more time spent on reading and doing mathematics. The Bible is a good book to incorporate into our children's daily reading. As parents, we must begin to guide their minds at an early age to keep them out of Satan's clutches. He has stolen so many of our young people's mind.

Parents should find ways to cut down on a lot of idle time and this will help keep them out of trouble. There is an old saying, "an idle mind is the devil's work shop." As parents, we need to keep our children's minds focused and occupied on positive things. We know if the enemy gets their minds, he has their whole body, and he is in total control. They become as puppets on a string with no mind at all. That's why it is important to start training our children and guiding their minds at early age. They are never too young to learn, because they are very smart at an early age. I have heard the statement made, "they don't know any better, they are babies." Yes, they do know better. They know more than what we give them credit for knowing. As parents, we just need to apply the instructions that have been given to us through God's Word. Again, even though children may stray away, they will return because a good foundation has been set.

There is a difference between obeying and honoring. Obey means to do as one is told; whereas honor means to respect and love. The Bible should be the guide we use to set the foundation for our children. The Word of God cannot and will not lead us wrong, because His Word is pure. We can bank on His Word, which will not fail and will never change. That's why we study God's Word daily so that it may be a constant reminder of the things that we should be doing. When you know to study and you refuse to do so, you miss out on a lot of important knowledge that was intended just for you. When we study the Word of God, we get to know Him in a more excellent way. We will become familiar with His voice and we will know when He is speaking and not the enemy. We must teach our children the importance of studying God's Word so that they can begin at an early age getting to know God for themselves. They will know what they should and should not do.

The Word of God teaches them to have an obedient spirit toward their parents and all adults. When they are told that they cannot do something and the answer is no, they will not go off the deep end. As parents, we must have do's and don'ts rules, for our children to abide by. Children should not be allowed to take over their parents' home. Parents should maintain control of their home at all times. No room in their home should be off limit to them. They should have access to every room in their home. Children should be made to understand that their parents' are always in charge.

CHAPTER FIVE:
PROPER EATING HABITS

We must begin to use proper eating habits and also teach our children to do the same. I realize that so many grown folks don't know how to eat properly. You should never pile up your plate with lots of food even if you are a big eater. You may want to take this thought into consideration, because you may be overindulging in food. This can only be corrected through self-control. For those of you, who do not eat much, begin with small portions of everything, and then if you desire more, you can go back for a second helping. One or two things will happen when someone over fills his or her plate. One, you will over eat or two a lot of food will be dumped into the garbage. I have seen both situations happen. That's not being considerate of someone who could have eaten what you wasted. I have seen it happen in homes, restaurants, and other functions where there is an all-you-can-eat buffet. This is my opinion: I feel that it's a sin to be wasteful.

I realize that many people have not given this any thought and there will continue to be many who will never give this any thought. Anything that becomes a habit, it appears to be all right to that person. We are creatures of habits. Any food that you are not sure about, you should get a small helping of that food. If you really like it, then go back and get more, and if you didn't like it, there is nothing wasted. You should never get a lot of anything, even when eating at home. This will cut out the wasting of food that maybe someone else could have eaten.

Proper eating habits will also help you maintain your weight or lose weight. Eating three basic meals and snacks during the course of a day will help you to lose weight and maintain a good weight. You will never lose weight by skipping meals or eating one large meal at the end of the day. The body stores up the food that you ate during that one meal, because it senses that you are not going to feed it regularly. This happens only when it becomes a pattern, and done over a long period of time. The body will pick up this irregular eating habit and begin to store up what you eat, which causes you not to lose the unnecessary weight.

Experts recommend that you eat breakfast, snack, lunch, snack, dinner, and snack in that order. Breakfast is the most important meal of the day, because the brain needs to be fed, it gives you energy. You should never allow yourself to become hungry unless, you are fasting for a period of time. Weight loss is harder when you starve yourself. While sometimes even though difficult, you must eat well balanced meals, regularly. Eating healthy meals will help you lose weight and maintain your weight. The right combination of food is very helpful in maintaining a well-balanced diet. Eating a healthy, balanced meal will correct many of our health issues over time.

A wholesome breakfast consist of eggs, oatmeal, grits, brown rice, toast (100% whole grain bread, not whole wheat), Cold cereals (100% whole grain), your choice of fruit, water, coffee (black is better or with a natural sweetener, Stevia), fruit juices (not from concentrate, no sugar added, no high fructose corn syrup), almond milk, rice milk, and coconut milk (not animals milk). These are your healthier choices of breakfast items. You may choose from any combination of these items to have a wholesome breakfast. For me, it is a bowl of oatmeal with raisins, cinnamon, and walnuts, two eggs, a banana, water and juice for most mornings. Occasionally, I will have something from the list below such as, biscuit, jelly, syrup, white rice, grits and bacon, which is in moderation. Water is the first thing that goes in my body in the morning; it is a purifier. Other breakfast items are: bacon (pork or turkey), sausage (pork or turkey). ham (pork or turkey), eggs, omelets, biscuits, toast, pancakes, white rice, grits, hash browns, jelly, jam, syrup, margarine or butter, juice, milk, coffee with sugar and cream, and cold cereals.

Changing the way we eat is a process; therefore, it does not mean that you have to cut out everything at once. By changing the way we eat, what we eat, and when we eat, we can eat ourselves back to good health. But, you should gradually cut back and cut out some things you are eating--that are not good for you. For example, processed foods (hot dogs, bologna, smoked sausages), and red meat (beef), unless you buy grass fed beef from a local farmer. Some things should only be eaten or drank in moderation. An expert from the internet explains, "Processed meats: In a 2013 study published in BMC Medicine, researchers concluded that of 26,344 deaths studied, high consumption of processed meat was responsible for 3.3 percent of them. Apart from being packed with preservatives and sodium, processed, packaged meats are high in nitrates, which have been linked to stomach cancer, says **Jim White, R D., spokesperson for the Academy of Nutrition & Dietetics and owner of Jim White Fitness training studios**. We must train our minds to focus on a healthier life style. You must begin by programming the mind that you are going to eat and drink healthier. The mind will get the message and begin to work with the body.

There are many things we can do to help the process of

healthy eating, which start with the chewing of our food. We must take the time to chew our food well before releasing it into our stomachs. Some foods should be chewed 10 or more times before releasing it. For example, your solid foods, meat, vegetables, fruits, nuts and bread. When you chew more, you will eat less. We must remember that we are not chickens: we cannot just swallow our food; therefore, we must chew because God blessed us with teeth to chew our food until very fine. By chewing more, eating the right food, and eating at the right time, we can eliminate health issues by spreading nutrients throughout the body. By eating the right food, you can eliminate medications and never have that medical issue again. Good health depends on how well you treat your body over time.

The body needs maintenance just like anything else. It needs up-keeping and nurturing in order to yield good health. You cannot treat your body any kind of way and expect it to serve you well. If you believe that, then you are in for a big let-down. As one expert explains, "Eliminate universal poisons. That includes nasty things like trans-fats, high-fructose corn syrup, artificial flavor and colors, and preservatives. But it can also include everyday ingredients like sugar and flour (since most flours act very much like sugars in the body)." By getting rid of these problematic foods, it can make a huge difference in your health, weight, and overall sense of wellbeing. You must begin by taking the time to check out the foods that you are consuming. Look at the food labels to check for sodium (salt), sugar, fat, cholesterol, high fructose corn syrup. These are things I look for when I am shopping for food, because many health issues stem from them. Checking these items while you shop will help you to determine whether to purchase an item or not. It is important to be aware of what you are consuming. Being familiar with food labels and the information they provide will make you aware, an informed consumer.

Food is appealing to the eyes and very tasteful to the taste buds, but the pleasure of eating should not take priority over eating right. The enemy makes everything look good and taste good. I have learned that everything that looks good and tastes good is not necessarily good for the body. As we learn better, we can make a conscience effort to do better by changing our lifestyle. This is the result of a disciplined approach for good health, and an effort to correct these health problems associated with our diet and condition of our body. God has given us the power to control our flesh through the Holy Spirit, but if we refuse to use the power within, then we are giving control to the flesh, which can cause a reversal of good health. God wants us to live by the power of the Holy Spirit that lives within each believer. The Scripture says, *"This I say then, walk in the Spirit, and you shall not fulfill the lust of the flesh"* (Galatians 5:16). God knows that the flesh is weak, but the Holy Spirit has power to over shadow the flesh. The flesh and the spirit tug against each other; therefore, they are contrary one to the other.

When we allow the Word of God through the Holy Spirit to penetrate our minds, we will begin to see the beauty of God's work in us. We will begin to seek godly things for our lives, our family, and others. We will begin to care about the environment in which we live. We will begin to seek those choices that are pleasing to Him. Paul says, *"Those things, which you have both learned, and received, and heard, and seen in me, do; and the God of peace shall be with you"* (Philippians 4:9). God will be with us at all times when we are in His will. If God is with us, He is able to keep our lives intact and also keep us from falling into temptation. God has the power to do just that and so much more.

God just wants you to have a sincere heart and He will do the rest. He wants you to be His dependent and totally depending on Him for all your needs and wants. The Scripture says, *"But my God shall supply all your needs according to His riches in glory by Christ Jesus"* (Philippians 4:19). God promised to supply all your needs, if you just trust and obey. If you have a need for healing, surely God can handle that need, you just have to acknowledge Him; with no reason to wonder if He will. You should trust that He can and He will keep His promises to His people. I have learned when I totally trust God to handle my situation, even though the problem still exists, God works it out when I least expect Him to do so. In other words, I do not dwell on the issue, but truly trust Him to handle the situation. You can certainly follow this pattern: pray, believe, and trust Him, as it concerns your health.

We put ourselves through unnecessary situations because we are holding on to worldly things and we are not truly seeking God's Will. God gave us a way to escape the lust of the flesh, and that is through the Holy Spirit who Jesus sent as our comforter, who leads, guides, and protects us. The Scripture says, *"Whither shall I go from thy Spirit? Or whither shall I flee from thy presence? If I ascend up into heaven, thou are there: if I make my bed in hell, behold, thou are there"* (Psalm 139:7-8). The Holy Spirit is ever present. If we allow the Holy Spirit to take charge of our lives, we will be able to with stand evil forces. When the Holy Spirit leads us, we will not submit to the flesh which causes us to disobey the Will of God. The Scripture says, *"And grieve not the Holy Spirit of God, whereby ye are sealed unto the day of redemption"* (Ephesians 4:30 KJV). The indwelling power of the Holy Spirit helps us to become more like Jesus each day, as we take on His characteristics of love and obedience.

We must remember that we were created to be governed by God's rules and regulations. According to the Word of God, *"For by Him were all things created, that are in heaven, and that are in the earth, visible and invisible, whether they be thrones, or dominions, or principalities, or powers: all things were created by Him and for Him: and He is before all things; and by Him all things consist"* (Colossians 1:16-17KJV). We belong to God, and we were created to serve God and should make Him our first priority. God doesn't need us because He owns everything; but we need Him, because we do not own anything: not even ourselves. Sometimes, I sit and think about how far we have come and how much God has given us. I am reminded of our ancestors who had very little, but they had a Big God, whom they trusted and followed. Most of them could not read or write, but they found ways to communicate with God.

Today, most of us have some form of education, but we are too busy or too lazy to read the Bible to communicate with God, or hear His guidance for our life. We have put everything before him. It hurts my heart when I see people acting in this manner. Even when we become alienated from His will, at some point in our lives, we should have enough sense to get back on track and in line with His Word. It's not necessary to spend the rest of our lives in the danger zone. Outside of the Will of God is a dangerous place to be, don't stay there! Return to God our first love; who waits patiently for us with open arms, but He will not wait forever. We do not want God's anger kindled against us, as it did toward the Israelites. He gave them warning after warning, through the prophets and spiritual leaders. Yet, they continued to disobey Him. God loved them dearly, but He got tired of pleading with them to repent and return back to Him. Let's not allow anything to become more important than God in our lives.

We sometimes allow our education and sophistication to stand in the way of our wisdom and knowledge of God. These things are good to have in place, but they are not the source of wisdom. I am a living witness that when you believe, have faith, and trust in God, He will take care of all of your needs. Education and sophistication are very important tools to have in your possession, but they don't supersede God in your life. Education and sophistication can only take you part of the way, but God can take you all the way to the top. In this case, it is definitely who you know and not what you know. The love of God can get you through some hard times. It is better to have God and no money than to have money and no God. Even though money is a good thing to have, God gives us the gifts and talents to make money: your money is connected to God. Money can be a cure for all things if we keep it in its proper perspective.

We do not want to be like the Israelites, who were hard hearted and a stiff-necked people. They refused to obey God's Word, repent of their sin, and return back to God. God's anger kindled against them and He wiped them out by the thousands. They were His chosen people, but they were very disobedient. The Scripture says, *"For the Lord said of them, they shall surely die in the wilderness. And there was not left a man of them, save Caleb the son of Jephunneh, and Joshua the son of Nun"* (Numbers 26:65). God wiped out the entire older generation. Caleb's and Joshua's lives were spared because they were obedient to their leader, Moses. Caleb and Joshua were part of the twelve spies that were sent by Moses to check out the land of Cana. They were the only two spies that came back with a good report, which was the truth; and the other ten spies came back with a bad report, which was false. The people decided to follow the spies who brought back a bad report, instead of following Caleb and Joshua who brought back a good report. After the death of Moses, God did not allow anyone to enter the Promised Land over the age of 20 except for Joshua and Caleb.

The younger generation of the Israelites entered the land that had been promised to them, after wandering in the wilderness for forty years. After losing their entire adult generation, the new generation was able to maintain its spiritual direction. God's Laws and spiritual character were still intact. A census was taken thirty-eight years earlier which showed over 600,000 men not including the women and children. The new census showed over 601,000 people that would enter the Promised Land. When it comes to the health situation, I see the same stiff-necked hard-hearted people who are determined to have things their way and not God's way. His way is the only way.

When I look at all of those people who were destroyed because of false information, I am reminded of today's society, who is being destroyed because of false information concerning their health. We are just like those people following the crowd and not the voice of God. Jesus talked about the "strait gate," and "narrow way" that leads to life, and the "wide gate," and the "broad way" that leads to destruction." The Scripture says, *"Enter ye in at the strait gate: for wide is the gate, and broad is the way, that lead to destruction, and many there be which go in there at: because strait is the gate, and narrow is the way, which lead unto life and few there be that find it"* (Matthew 7:13-14). Jesus gives us a choice; it is up to us to choose the right one. As it relates to food, it is up to us to choose the right food for our bodies. We are always looking at the bigger broader picture in life, but small narrow things hold more value.

The ten spies caused a whole generation of people to be destroyed, because of false information, fear and lack of faith. The Israelites got caught up in what they could see right then, and not what God had already done, the things He had already brought them through. The people got to the last step, but refused to take it, because they stopped trusting God. We too are like the Israelites, trusting God to handle the small things, but doubting His ability to handle the big problems. It is like we are saying to Him, God, I trust you to keep a roof over my head, clothes on my back, food on my table, provide transportation and put gas in my car, but I don't trust You to help me discipline myself, to control my eating habits to lose weight. I trust the doctors and medicine to control high blood pressure, diabetes, strokes, cancer, kidney disease, high cholesterol, heart disease, without even thinking about the power God has given us. According to Luke, *"Behold, I give unto you power to tread on serpents and scorpions, and over all the power of enemy: and nothing shall by any means hurt you"* (Luke 10:19). God gives us power over serpents and scorpions that can harm us.

Today, I am speaking to Christian people (believers); we are the ones who should know better. I don't expect the unsaved people to have faith and trust in God, He is not their Father. Satan is their father, and some of them are in better health condition than we are. God's Word holds the truth which is our Bibles, but we are looking for answers from every source, except the Bible. God has given us every tool we need in His Word, to fix all that ails us. We are so laid back with our current situations that nothing seems to faze us. What I see is a whole generation of people being wiped out by poor food choices, bad eating habits, smoking, drinking, and drugging. What will it take for God's people to step up and take control of their health?

God will bring His judgment upon those who continue to disobey His Word. God will not allow us to continue in our sin and continue to ignore Him. God brought judgment against the Israelites because of their disobedience. The Scripture says, *"And the LORD said unto Moses, How long will this people provoke me and how long will it be before they believe me, for the signs for which I have done among them I will smite them with the pestilence, and disinherit them, and will make of thee a greater nation and mightier than they"* (Numbers 14:11-12). He will destroy everything that we touch until we come to our senses, repent and turn back to Him. We need God's help in everything we do. We need Him to guide us in every decision that we make. We need to always consult with Him before we make major decisions, because God knows what is best for us. We must be like David who never made any decision without first consulting with God. He knew he could count on God to receive the right answer.

The help of God is permanent; everything else temporary and will only last a season. There are people who put their trust in wealth, jobs, cars, houses, careers, and families. These things are temporary and none of them can heal our bodies or give us peace within: only God can. When God is our first priority, He will keep us abreast of everything that we need to know, about our mind, body and soul, which is the total man. We must remember that everything we do can be viewed as seasons which only last for a period of time.

CHAPTER SIX:
THE FOUR SEASONS OF LIFE

I see life as seasons: spring, summer, fall, and winter. There is a season for everything under the sun. The Scripture states, *"To everything there is a season, and a time to every purpose under the heaven"* (Ecclesiastes 3:1). Every season has a purpose in our life and must function in its' own time frame. Spring is the season when things come to life, and begin to grow. I see people's lives the same way. From birth to twenty-five, we are in the growing stage of life. This is a season for trials and errors. We also make many foolish decisions in life during this season. Most of the time, young people are not serious about anything; not even life. Everything is really cool. At that age, our minds are being molded and shaped as we mature. This season is where children need to be introduced to healthy food. Then, there is summer which is from twenty-six to fifty. At that stage, life is in full blossom at that age and maturity begins to settle in. We should be making sound decisions and wise choices in life. We should be making better food choices at this stage of life. Next, there is fall which is from fifty-one to seventy-five. Life should have reached full maturity by this age. Things are gradually changing during the fall. We will begin to reap the benefit of good Health from our food choices. Finally, there is winter which is from seventy-six to death. We know that winter is usually the season where life comes to an end on earth. Food choices we made in the previous seasons determine our body functions.

As Christians, we must strive for maturity to begin making better decisions and choices in life earlier in our life seasons. As we grow into maturity, we should make decisions and choices based on knowledge and wisdom. It's sad when you find Christians who have not gotten past the milk stage in life. Like babies, they are still adapting to solid food. They have become stagnated which means they have stop growing. They have become complacent and stuck, which is not good for anyone. As long as there is life in our bodies, we should make a conscience effort to strive for perfection. Even though there is none perfect except for the Father, we should strive to get as close as possible, to perfection like Christ. Each day that God allows us to see, should motivate us to do better than the day before. We should never want to stop growing. When I awake in the morning, I realize that I have been blessed to see a new day. I'm excited about another chance to do something that I didn't do the day before. The fact that somebody didn't get up to see a new day, motivates me to be a better person than I was the day before; with each new dawn, God has given us another opportunity to get right whatever we messed up the day before. As Christians, we must continue to grow in God's grace.

Spring time (ages 0 to 25) is also the season where parents play a major role in their children's lives. They set the tone for their children and direction for their future. We are their first role model. Parents are obligated to set good examples for their children to follow, as well as introduce them to the Word of God. As parents, we should live godly lives before our children. Parents are caretakers for their children, because God has placed them in our care; therefore, we must take care of them in a godly way. As parents, we do not have the right to neglect our children nor deprive them of a wholesome life. In order to build a quality relationship with our children, we must spend quality time with our children. They did not ask to come here. It was by our choice that they are here whether it was planned or unplanned. We are obligated to honor our responsibility for our children's sake. Children observe everything their parents do. If they never see anything positive in our lives, they will not have anything positive to base their lives upon. If they see only negative things of life, they are more likely to make bad choices with health, and their life.

Next, there is the summer season (ages 25 to 50) where everything is continuing to grow toward maturity. Summer is when everything is in full blossom. There are many shade trees, flowers, and green grass. Everything is growing to a more mature stage in life. After going through the immaturity stage, children's lives begin to form and shape into the adulthood. During this season, parents begin to step back and allow their children to be tested and experience life on their own. This is the season that will make or break young people. In this season, young adults begin to focus more on the important things in life. They will continue to grow until they reach the maturity stage. Of course, the road is rocky along the way, but if they remain steadfast in the LORD, know and understand the source of their help. It is good to know where all of your help come from. According to Psalm, *"I will lift up mine eyes unto the hills, from whence cometh my help. My help cometh from the Lord, which made heaven and earth"* (Psalm 121:1-2). If a solid foundation has been set in the Lord, they will survive.

Then, there is the fall season (ages 50 to 75) where everything has grown to maturity and is ready to be harvested, also, set aside for seed time for the next growth season. Life can be viewed in this same manner. When people reach maturity according to age, they are able to apply the wisdom and knowledge gained, in their early seasons are more ready to settle down and focus on the godly things of life. In the spiritual realm, we continue to mature, until we cross over to the other side. We begin to put away childish things and focus more on a God kind of life. The Scripture says, *"The days of our years are threescore years and ten; and if by reason of strength they be fourscore years, yet is their strength labor and sorrow; for it is soon cut off and we fly away"* (Psalm 90:10 KJV). We should be making plans for a healthy and prosperous life as we journey through this season. Fall is the season where things are changing and the leaves are falling from the trees.

The life of a Christian may be viewed in the same manner as the fall season. Throughout the growth cycle, we continue to peel off sin and excess baggage from our lives. It bothers me to see people who are over fifty still making foolish decisions and allowing the enemy to use them, just for a few moments of pleasure. You would think by this time, we would have matured enough to build on a solid foundation and not walk on such shaky ground. You are over the hill, and you are not going backward, but forward. Most of the time, we have convinced ourselves that we still have time to make changes, to get it right, but we don't have the time that we believe we have. Why would anyone want to continue to make foolish decisions when it comes to their life or their health? We can keep on saying we are going to get ourselves together, but until we exercise will power to get ourselves together, we must rely upon God's power through the Holy Spirit, to keep us straight and on the narrow path.

Finally, the winter season (ages 75 to death) is where we enter our most mature stage of life. This is where we should be wise, have plenty of wisdom, and much knowledge of God's Word, and His way. When we think of the winter season, we think of cold, dark and dreary days, often very uncomfortable. As Christians, we should not be concerned about those days, but we should continue to look forward to the bright and warm days of life. During this season, heaven should be our main goal. If we are blessed, by the time we reach our winter season, we should have put away all the foolish things of life, and have made preparation for our eternal destiny. Winter is where things die and life comes to a close here on earth. As believers in Christ, we will have eternal life. The Scripture says, *"Let not your heart be troubled; ye believe in God, believe also in me. In my Father's house are many mansions: if it were not so, I would have told you. I go to prepare a place for you. And if I go and prepare a place for you, I will come again, and receive you unto myself; that where I am, there ye may be also"* (John 14:1-3). Jesus has promised eternal life for all believers. If we prepare for the winter season during the other seasons, we could have warm, bright, and beautiful sun shining days. We, ourselves play a major role in how well our winter season will be. It is determined by the lifestyle we have lived and how well we have cared for our bodies. This is why, it is important to live a God kind of life.

CHAPTER SEVEN:
ANOTHER HEALTH ISSUE –
MENOPAUSE / HOT FLASHES

Menopause is an issue that has been labeled many things. I have heard all types of stories about menopause or going through the change, as older women termed this issue. Some of them freaked out over this ordeal, thought they were losing their mind, because they did not understand what was going on with their bodies. In all things, get an understanding, in every situation. The Scripture says, *"Wisdom is the principal thing; therefore get wisdom: and with all thy getting get an understanding"* (Proverbs 4:7). Mostly, understanding is the key to a healthier lifestyle. Menopause is the simple act of making a transitional change from, having a cycle, to not having a cycle (menstrual period). When women reach a certain age, they stop having a cycle, though not at the same age. Some women will stop early in life and others will stop later in life. It does not have anything to do with hot flashes or night sweats. I know some young women who are having hot flashes. Hot flashes can be caused by a numbers of things, such as certain food items, (example) beverages, or simply how well we take care of our bodies when we are young. In other cases, medications, and vaginal surgery, such as a hysterectomy contributes to hot flashes. Some of it is a belief that has been passed down from generations to generations. God always gives somebody the knowledge to correct things that are myth and are not true.

I thank God for allowing me get a handle on this situation. I never experienced any of the symptoms that I had heard about, nor changes in my body or body function. When I hear other women speaking about certain situations going on with their bodies, I can't relate. I have never experienced back pain, and aching joints due to arthritis. I have always been very active, and I have pretty much eaten healthy foods, like vegetables, fruits, beans and nuts. I learned in my youth how to take care of my temple that God entrusted in my care. I ate wholesome foods, exercised and now I am reaping the benefits of doing it the right way. I am 68 and still active. When you have gained good knowledge, you should utilize it to your benefit. I realize that women have different needs and our bodies are different which is why I encourage every woman to get to know her own body, her needs, and her family history. A woman armed with this information can control many of the health issues facing us today like symptoms of menopause, weight gain, bodily aches and pains.

The Holy Spirit has allowed me to observe people eating certain food or drinking certain beverages---how they reacted after they finished consuming these items. They have lots of sugar and caffeine with the above items I mentions earlier. A small item like a stick of gum has too much sugar for some people. Christmas 2008, I baked many sweets and I had a sweets party. After consuming a piece of every sweet throughout the day, I went to bed and I awoke in the middle of the night, drenched with sweat. The Holy Spirit brought to my attention immediately all the sweets that I had consumed during the day. He allowed me to experience these same symptoms to show me what happens when I over indulge in a lot of sweets. This is my own personal testimony of the effect many sweets can have on the body. An expert from the internet, Dr. Christiane Northrup explains, "Hot flashes occur when blood vessels in the skin of the head and neck open more widely than usual allowing more blood to shift into the area, creating heat and redness. Researchers believe that the Vascular shift due to changes in neurotransmitter activity that are not fully understood, occur in response to erratic hormone level" (www.drnorthrup.com). When too much sugar and caffeine gets in blood vessels, it rushes to the brain. The brain reacts, which causes the sweat to begin to pour out of the body almost immediately.

Normally, sweets may be eaten with a meal, and in moderation, except for those people with medical conditions, which exclude sugar from their diet, you should be ok. We get in trouble with anything when we over indulge. God knew I needed to experience these symptoms in order to be able to write about this issue. What we consume is the cause of many of our health issues and problems. I have not had that situation to occur again, because I watch my sugar intake, added more fruit to my diet, I do not over indulge in any area. What I usually do is to go four days without eating any sweets, or having any sugar, and on the weekend, I will treat myself to something sweet. Even if sweets are one of your weaknesses, exercising and discipline will allow you to treat yourself without over indulging.

One Sunday afternoon, I was waiting in the Friendship Hall of our church. One of my sisters came in with a cup of coffee, and as soon as she finished that cup of coffee, she got hot, and sweat started rolling down her face. She began to fan. The Holy Spirit allowed me to see that incident so I could better understand hot flashes. There were two things that could have caused the hot flashes: the sugar and the caffeine in the coffee. From my observing other people and my own experience, too much sugar is a known factor in contributing to hot flashes. An expert from the internet, Dr. Christine Northrup lists some things that contribute to hot flashes, such as foods we consume, "Sugar, caffeine, and how women in south American and Mexico have only a 10 percent rate of hot flashes and menopauses" (www.drnorthrup.com). As you begin to work toward better health, use less sugar and caffeine in your diet and see immediate results. Because of the hidden sugar in processed foods and caffeine in the diet, there are so many ways that people can get sugar and caffeine. Educating ourselves by reading food label to find out what is in our food. Articles about food nutrition can lead to healthier life style.

While writing this book, I read many articles. This article from an expert explains, "This story reminded me that just as nursing a baby is affected by what its mother eats because it is passed to the baby through their mother's milk, we are affected by the foods and drinks that we put in our bodies. There is a wealth of great advice about how to deal with the symptoms of menopause, but you don't hear much about how food can be our greatest ally in combating our menopause symptoms. Certain foods can calm us or make us more irritable or simply push us off-balance. Through working with thousands of women, we've observed that certain foods and drinks do seem to bring on hot flashes and night sweats, while others work well to subdue them, according to Marcelle Pick, OB/GYN NP"

www.womentowomen.com./menopause-perimenopause/nutritional-relief- for-hot-flashes/

Foods and drinks play a major role in our health issues.

Changing the way we eat can make a big difference in how healthy we are and how well we feel. My argument is that hot flashes are not linked to menopause. I believe one has nothing to do with the other. I want to clear up that myth. I have heard many horrible stories about menopause that does not hold true, I am living proof. To be honest, I don't believe there is any such thing as menopause. This is another one of those myths that man came up with, which can't be found in God's Word. The Bible mentions old age and how we should grow old gracefully. I am reminded of Abraham and Sarah who had a child in their old age. He was a hundred and she was ninety. Surely she was not going through menopause, according to man's definition. I feel good health is all in how well you take care of yourself as you are getting older.

I am not the only one; there are women in other countries that have no knowledge of the words "hot flashes" or the word "menopause". These are foreign words for them, but for us, we believe it's a way of life. They have not heard of these symptoms because they are eating the right kinds of food. They are not eating a lot of junk, such as sugar, salt, bad fat, artificial sweeteners, and taking pills. They use the real food that Mother Nature provides for them. America is the queen of sugar, salt, processed foods and pills. We are flashing everywhere, and we don't think anything about what is going on with our bodies. For us, this is the norm---we have our own personal name for hot flashes "private summer". What we fail to realize is that hot flashes are a sign that there is something irregular going on within our bodies, and most of the time, the cause is the food that we consume. Mother Nature has provided for us the best medicine cabinet on earth which is our vegetables, fruits, berries and nuts all natural foods. Mother Nature has designed a vegetable or a fruit, for every sickness and every disease. If you put enough vegetables and fruits in your body, they will block the diseases and keep them from attacking your body. As one expert from Prevention Remedies explains, "Researchers have discovered that healthy foods are the best medicine for the human body and not pills". Instead of spending our money wisely, such as investing in healthy foods, we would rather spend it on medication. We have been made to believe that a pill is better than natural food. What's in a small pill that would cause it to be more effective than a well-balanced meal? Anything that is quick and easy, we jump on right away. It appears for some, they are waiting for the opportunity to start popping pills.

I am so grateful to God for giving me wisdom and knowledge to know and understand that menopause is a transitional change in the female body and not some life threatening health issue. Even though I have heard many horrible stories about menopause, I learned that they were just false information, due to a lack of understanding. When my cycle stopped, I did not experience any major changes as far as life. I continued to do everything that I had been doing, before my cycle stopped. One good thing came out of that ordeal. My blood count went up and I have not experience being anemic any more. Throughout my life, anemia and low blood pressure were my biggest health issues. I can remember when I would lose my sight, get dizzy and not be able to see, which only lasted for a few minutes, I never allowed those issues to get me down. I kept right on moving. Sometimes, when I would visit my doctors for a checkup, they didn't understand how I was able to do all the things I did, because my blood count would be so low. But, I know, that it was the grace of God that kept me going. According to the Scripture, *"Thou will keep him in perfect peace, whose mind is stayed on thee: because he trusts in thee"* (Isaiah 26:3). The Scripture says I will have perfect peace, if I keep my mind on God. I will be able to block the devil's false information, which he tries to put in my mind concerning my health. Most health issues stem from the things that we are consuming that are bad for us, and also from the neglect of things that we should be consuming that are good for us. By changing the way we eat, we can correct many of our health issues, over time.

I am so grateful to God for giving me wisdom and

understanding to know that everything man predicts is not the truth. When my doctor suggested that I should start taking hormones pills, I refused. My God said my body is fearfully and wonderfully made. According to the Scripture, "I will praise thee; for I am fearfully and wonderfully made: marvelous are thy works; and that my soul knows right well" (Psalm 139:14). If God's Word is true, and I believe it is, I do not have to rebuild my body; just take care of what I have been given. The body requires maintenance, done the natural way, and not with a bunch of pills. I have a great body, and there is no swelling, puffiness, and bloating. God has a natural plan for our bodies through Mother Nature. I was watching TV one day, and there were two doctors on a talk show who were discussing menopause. They were talking about the issues women face when they go through menopause, and how the body changes. I sat there and listened, and could not relate to anything they said, because I have not experienced any of those symptoms. There were women who were taking hormone pills, asked the doctors how long to take the pills. There were some who have been on the pills for many years. One doctor advised it depends on the woman, and what her body requires. Some women need hormone pills for a short time, and others longer. The other doctor advised taking hormone pills should not exceed five years. I was observing the weight of those women, and would be willing to stake my life that they have some other health issues going, in their bodies. As I stated before, many of our health issues can be corrected just by changing our lifestyle.

CHAPTER EIGHT:
CONSULT GOD BEFORE
MAKING HEALTH DECISIONS

In the early 70's, I was diagnosed with fibroid tumors. At that time, they were the size of a dime. They were so small that my doctor said there was no reason for concern at that time. I had no idea that certain foods made them grow. Had I known, I probably would have changed my eating habits then. I don't know that for sure, because I did not have the wisdom, knowledge, and understanding that I have now. By the latter part of the 80's, several tumors had grown to the size of an orange, and I began to experience heavy bleeding. My doctor became concerned and recommended that I have surgery. I was at the beauty shop one day and I picked up a magazine to read. There was an article that mentioned women who were diagnosed with fibroid tumors. The article stated, "Ninety percent of women who have a hysterectomy did not need it." In other words, there are other methods that can treat these symptoms.

I began to do some research on my own. I learned that the hysterectomy was a quick fix and that's why doctors recommend that type of surgery. I have since learned that this type of surgery is not in the best interest of women. I have spoken to women who have had a hysterectomy, and who said that they wish they had used another alternative. In other words, they have encountered other problems since their surgery. After the surgery, a woman's body has to be reconstructed as much as possible to compensate for what has been removed from her body. This is typically done through medication, which causes other side effects. Hot flashes are one of the side effects caused by hormone medication. I am so grateful to God for allowing me to hold out and not take the easy way out. By trusting God, I was able to beat the odds that were against me. That's why it is so important to trust God in everything we do, because He knows what is best for us.

I began to educate myself on fibroid tumors by visiting Champion's Pharmacy in Memphis, TN (Website: www.theherbalman.com), where I found lots of information on fibroids. The information included the type of teas to drink, food to eat and the food not to eat in order for them to shrink. I worked not far from the pharmacy and would spend my lunch break at the pharmacy, looking for information on fibroid tumors. I was able to gather lots of materials on fibroid tumors, such as, pamphlets and articles. I read one article where a woman who had fibroid tumors never had surgery, because she changed her eating habits. There were certain foods she cut out of her diet. She explained how certain foods made the tumors grow like potato chips, fried foods, and sweets. The fatty foods caused them to grow. After reading her story, I began to follow that same pattern by watching the food that I was eating, and it paid off. Just a little bit of discipline changed my life situation.

By listening to the Holy Spirit, I was able to save myself from having major surgery. I am so grateful to God for helping, leading, and guiding me in the right direction. Again, it pays to trust God and not man, because God has the answer to every situation. I asked God to heal my body, and He did. The Scripture says, *"Ask, and it shall be given you; seek, and ye shall find; knock, and it shall be opened unto you: for every one that asks receives; and he that seeks finds; and to him that knocks it shall be opened"* (Matthew 7:7-8). We must have patience to wait on God to deliver. If He said it; He's going to do it. We should not give up on God. We must continue to be persistent in our asking.

God directed me to the right source; I was able to change my eating habits and not having to have surgery. I am so grateful to God for that. I began buying the herb teas and I was drinking about four different teas every day. Champion's Pharmacy has what it calls a fibroid kit that you can purchase that contains all the recommended teas. I would get up very early to make sure I had enough time to drink the teas before I went to work. I did this for four years, and by the grace of God, I was able to eliminate the surgical option. Herbs are natural and are good for the body. It was a slow process, but they did shrink enough for me to endure them during my healing. At that time, I still had a cycle which fibroids can feed on the blood flow and continue to grow. After my cycle stopped, thank God I had no more problems with fibroid tumors! I have since learned that a good source of vitamin D-3 will also cause fibroid to shrink. There is a lot of information out there on fibroid, you just have to research. Do your research before you say yes to life altering surgery.

It always pays to let God guide your thought, and help you with your decision making. I am so thankful to God that I did not make a hasty decision. That's why it pays to never put your life in the hands of man, but always put your life in the hands of your maker, the Creator of life. Who would have better knowledge about your body than the One who made it? I could have taken the easy way out by having the surgery done, which is a quick fix, but with the potential for many new health issues. I am so glad that I listened to my heart and not the urgency of doctors who were encouraging me to have surgery at the time. After I refused to have the surgery, my doctors recommended that I have tests done to make sure the tumors were not cancerous. Each test came back negative for cancer. I thanked God for leading and directing me not to have the surgery, and eliminating the need to take hormone replacements. By God's grace and mercy, I have never had any type of major surgery and I don't see any major surgery in my future. I will continue to take care of my body, which is God's temple. The Scripture says, *"Know ye not that ye are the temple of God, and that the Spirit of God dwelleth in you? If any man defile the temple of God, him shall God destroy; for the temple of God is holy, which temple ye are"* (1 Corinthians 3:16-17). That is just one example of what can happen, when we take control of our health.

God is allowing me to write this book to shed some light on certain health issues. No, I am not a doctor, but I am writing under the unction of the Holy Spirit, and what the Spirit guides me to write; therefore, I am writing under the anointing of the Holy Spirit. The Holy Spirit promised to teach me all things. He prompted me to write this book to help the younger generation get a grip on health issues that plagued their ancestors. I want to let them know that they don't have to go through what their ancestors have gone through. The younger generation can break the generational curses by taking care of their bodies and changing their eating habits. Remember, we are what we eat! Fruits and vegetables should always be part of our daily meal. Certain fruits and vegetables can protect your body from many of the diseases that attack our bodies. These foods are called blockers. There is an old saying, "An apple a day will keep the doctor away." The simple fact of eating an apple everyday can work wonders for our bodies. The apple is one of my favorite fruits. I have cravings for apples and other fruits. My body has become accustomed to eating certain fruits daily. When I am running low on fruits, I know it's time to make a trip to the grocery store. I will elaborate on some of the other fruits and vegetables that are a good source of prevention.

Poor eating habits can cause major health problems such as, obesity, high blood pressure, diabetes, stroke, heart disease, cancer, and high cholesterol. There are others, but these are the most common ones. I have never seen so many ill people, and the hospitals are running over with ill people. When one patient is dismissed, another patient is waiting for that bed, and the hospitals are over-crowded. I wonder to myself sometimes, why are there so many sick people. There has to be an answer, but it does not seem to matter. Not to mention the mentally ill population, I had no idea we had so many mentally ill people until I started to work for Whitehaven Mental Health Center in 1984. Next, there is no end to the prescription drugs. Taking pills has become a way of life. We take pills in the morning and take pills at night before we go to bed. I am going to do everything in my power and that is humanly possible to ensure I do not become a part of the pill statistics. I am going to prove to the people of God that you can live a wholesome life, without pills. I know I can do just that with the help of God. The Scripture tells me that all things are possible through Christ. I am going to take God at His Word, and trust Him, to make it possible for me to live a drug free life.

Our doctors know that if we change the way we eat, we can eliminate the use of most medications. Their fear is that we are not disciplined enough to make the necessary changes. They are right, because most people do not want to put forth any effort to better their circumstances. That's why doctors continue to prescribe more and more medication. It is so sad how people are being brain washed into taking medication for fear of having a stroke or heart attack. The truth is; you could have a stroke or heart attack while taking medication. People are fearful of dying, but what they fail to realize is that God controls life and death.

The news media has begun to speak out concerning the

abuse of prescription drugs. You take a pill for one health problem and end up with more pills to take, and new health issues that stemmed from the first pill. We can change our eating habits and eliminate medication, because Mother Nature has designed things that way. We have got to start listening to the voice of the Holy Spirit and allowing Him to lead and direct our path, when it comes to our health. Who knows better than God about our health? My son, Dennis was diagnosed with diabetes in 2011, and immediately, he had to take insulin. He changed his eating habits for the better. He gave up bread, sweets, rice and he exercised daily. Just by disciplining himself to eat right and exercise, he was healed from diabetes. He no longer has diabetes and he does not take any medications. He is a living testimony that it can be done. We have to make a choice, whether to take pills for the rest of our lives or to eat the foods that can help us stay drug free. Yes, we can eat ourselves back to good health.

This can be done by eating the right combination of foods to get the body back on track. The American people have access to so much until we over indulge in everything. We are a country of plenty, of privileges, which is often abused and misused. I often think about people in other countries who are dying from malnutrition because of a lack of nutritious food. In America, people are dying from gluttony (habitual greed or excess in eating) Oxford Dictionaries. The Scripture says, *"Listen, my child be wise and give serious thought to the way you live. Don't associate with people who drink too much wine, or stuff themselves with food. Drunkards and gluttons will be reduced to poverty. If all you do is eat and sleep, you will soon be wearing rags"* (Proverbs 22:19-21 GNBV). There are so many people who are addicted to food; their lives are centered around food, unable to focus on anything else in life. Food is a wonderful thing when consumed in the proper manner, and harmful to your overall health when consumed improperly. I write this book as a wake- up call to those who are falling by the way side, when it comes to food. Food is like fire; it can work both ways. It can be good for you and it may be harmful for you if used incorrectly. The fact is that you have strength, or gain the strength needed to control bad eating habits, through the Holy Spirit.

Once, I read a story on the internet about a young man, who had a serious weight problem. He began to gain weight rapidly, at an early age. By the time he reached age eighteen, he was up to five hundred pounds. He did not stop there. He continued to gain weight, and by the time he was twenty-three, he was up to seven hundred ninety-nine pounds. One day after becoming very frustrated, he realized that he was between life and death. If he didn't do something about his weight, he would die. He became frightened and started to pray for strength to lose the weight. He knew he was going to die if he didn't change his life style. Little by little, he began to exercise, just standing up and sitting back down. As time went by, he was able to do more. He changed his eating habits, and began eating smaller portions of food. By the grace of God, he was able to lose five hundred pounds, without surgery or any diet supplements. He did it the natural way and of course it was not easy. He admitted that it was a struggle, but by the grace of God, he was able to endure the pain and suffering. Now, he is reaping the benefits of a healthy life style. He feels very good about his accomplishment. He admits that food is his number one fan, but he has learned to control it and not let it control him.

God keeps me in good health without any medication, and I know He can do the same for you. I refuse to contaminate God's Temple with a bunch of junk. I trust Him to keep me healthy, providing that I do my part to maintain a healthy life style. When I say to people that I don't take any medication, they look at me strange as if I should be taking some type of medication because of my age. When I say I don't take any medication, I mean absolutely nothing at all, prescription drugs or over-the-counter drugs. I have faith in God that He is who He says He is, and I trust Him to do what He said He would do. God wants us to prosper and be in good health. I say to people, we trust God or we don't trust Him; there is no in between. We must begin to take the word of God for what it is, because it will never change. The truth of the matter is; we can bank on the Word of God which cannot lie. The time has come, whereas we must allow the Word of God to have control over our lives, so that we can reap the full, matchless benefits of God's Blessings.

Healthcare is a major issue in today's society: the provision of good care, loss of good care, and the personal responsibility for seeking good health. It seems, as a whole, our nation is suffering from some form of health crisis. That deficiency has to be linked to something. Is it possible that some of our crises may be caused by sin? If you study the minor and major prophets, you will see instances where God destroyed whole nations because of their sin. They were disobedient to God's Word, refused to repent and turn from their wicked ways, and were therefore destroyed. God has always sent prophets to warn the people of their sin consequences and impending judgments. But, as is often the case, the people were self-centered, full of self-pride and ignored all warning signs. Could this be true of the personal health crises we are faced with today? Blood pressure, aches, pains, diabetes, and cholesterol are all warning signs from the body that something is amiss. God sends warning by spiritual leaders, before judgment. Early warning signs are meant to be heeded, and advice sought to prevent further damage. We must begin to listen with ears of faith to hear from God. God is such a loving, merciful and kind God, that He puts people in place to inform us, who truly care for your well-being, like me. I want God's people to be healthy. Don't be like 'most' people and continue in sin and drift into disease. Noah tried to warn the people, they laughed and scorned him, and said he must be losing his mind, because he was building a boat on dry land. Noah had received instruction from God, and he was being obedient to God's commands. He did not question God or ask why He was having him build the boat on dry land. Noah could have taken the same approach as most people, but he trusted God, and lived a long, prosperous life.

We should have that same mentality as Noah when it comes to the Word of God. Sometimes people are unsure what to believe or do. They know they have not been obedient and are not living according to the Word of God. I often look at Biblical examples of obedience and healing. For instance, the woman with the issue of blood was seeking medical help in all of the wrong places. She had suffered for twelve long years and spent her life savings trying to find a cure for her disease. The Scripture says, *"And a woman, which was diseased with an issue of blood twelve years, came behind Him, and touched the hem of His garment: for she said within herself, If I may but touch His garment, I shall be made whole"* (Matthew 9:20-21). It was not until she was able to touch the hem of Jesus' garment that her situation changed. But she had enough faith and trust to believe that one touch was all she needed to be healed. Sometimes, that one special touch from Jesus is all we need to change our situation. We cannot physically touch the hem of His garment, but we have access to His power through His Word. People are spending their life savings on healthcare and prescription drugs trying to get well, when all they need is a touch from Jesus which is through His Word. They are looking for help in all the wrong places. The Scripture says, *"But seek ye first the kingdom of God, and His righteousness; and all these things shall be added unto you"* (Matthew 6:33 KJV).

We have everything we need through the access of God's Word, but we are looking to man to solve our health issues and problems. Since we can't see God, we don't trust Him to solve our health issues and problems.

We have to use our imaginary mind and see God in everything and every situation. We realize that there are some things that only God can fix and solve, because He has all power. Man's power is limited and there are many things he does not have the capability to resolve. And yes, God does use man as an overseer of the earth, but man does not control the earth. We as a people give man power that he does not have knowledge to use. When we put our trust in God, He will give us the wisdom and knowledge to take care of our own health issues and problems, and guide us when faced with man's solutions, which are often monetary in nature.

The problems that I see when it comes to our health issues are lack of knowledge, which stems from not being educated on health issues. The proposed health solutions are either surgical or drug based, both costly alternatives. Whether it works or not, the fact is that the dollar amount for the prescription has already been collected. It is not only wise, but recommended that every patient do some research on the drugs being prescribed before agreeing to take them. No sense in being a voluntary guinea pig and conduct self-experimentation. Some prescription drugs can do more harm than good to our bodies over time. Seek second and third opinions if necessary before consuming new medication, to make sure that they are suitable, for your body and your condition.

I have heard enough stories about prescription drugs that I never want to put any in my body. I look at long term goals, how to stay healthy and live a prosperous life. Some people are living just for the moment. What we fail to realize is that our bodies become dependent on these drugs for survival. When I look at all the people that are on prescription drugs, this is not God's intention for healing. People are caught up in the prescription shuffle, and are not concerned about health issues. Sickness and disease are on the rise and no one seems to care enough about what it may take to change this pattern. It seems as if it is a no-win situation. People are acting as if this pattern is the norm, but I am just old enough to know that this is not the norm. There is an attack on our health, and the answer is found in the Word of God. The Scripture says, *"If my people, which are called by my name, shall humble themselves, and pray, and seek my face, and turned from their wicked ways; then will I hear from heaven, and forgive their sin, and will heal their land"* (2 Chronicles 7:14 KJV). We can change our health issues by submitting to God's request.

Part of Jesus' mission was to heal the sick, deaf, mute, blind and lame. The mission has not changed; the time is now for the Saints to step up and take a stand and continue Jesus' healing mission. If the Saints are ill, afflicted and diseased, how will the mission continue? We, as Christians, cannot allow the enemy to drag us down, through sickness and disease. The Scripture says, *"Is any among you afflicted let him pray. Is any merry Let him sing psalms. Is any sick among you let him call for the elders of the church; and let them pray over him, anointing him with oil in the name of the Lord: and the prayer of faith shall save the sick, and the Lord shall raise him up; and if he has committed sins, they shall be forgiven him"* (James 5:13-15). This passage was written by James, the brother of Jesus. He did not say call the doctors, but the elders who are called by God to take care of sick. Christians are to do a greater work than Christ did while He was here on earth.

Saints must let Satan know who we are, and that we are not going to bow down to him. We have been equipped with power to put Satan on notice. We have been given the power to continue the mission that Jesus started. As Saints, we can take back what Satan has stolen from God's people, such as peace, joy, happiness, good health, and a sound mind. First, we should take care of our own situations, of restoring our own good health and peace of mind, before taking care of someone else's health situations. Now, I understand why the work of the Saints have not always been effective, we have not faithfully used our God given power to take care of our own health and problems. It is the same precept as the flight attendant who teaches on safety. In other words, you take care of yourself first, before attempting to take care of someone else's need.

God warns us about all of the evil deeds that Satan will be doing in the last days here on earth. Sickness and diseases are not happening by accident. They are a part of the devils' plan to keep God's people bound and constricted. He knows there are certain things that we are addicted to and become slaves. Satan baits the hook and waits for us to bite, because he knows some people are vulnerable. We are addicted to so many things: food, tobacco, alcohol, drugs, sex, and more. These are the enemy's most powerful baits that he uses to trap us. We all know that food is good for the body, but when we become addicted to food and over indulge we take good things and turn them into bad things. Sex can be very good and healthy for the body, but should only take place between a husband and a wife according to the Bible. You have husbands and wives who get caught up in the cheating game which is another one of Satan's trap. Then, you have the single people who are shacking and have no remorse or shame. Sex in many instances has become such a violent act and has dire, unhealthy consequences. Alcohol is not a bad thing when done in moderation and as part of social gatherings. It becomes bad when you allow it to control you and you start to act like a foolish person. When it comes to tobacco and drugs, my prayer is that one day these "health hazards" will be eliminated totally from your body and our society. Not just the street drugs, but prescription drugs too and the list goes on.

CHAPTER NINE:
GETTING TO KNOW
YOUR UNIQUE BODY

God made every person a different body, even though we are each made in His image. Our glorious bodies operate the same, but have a unique genetic make-up. In order to control certain health issues we must get to know how our body functions when all is well. We come in all shapes, sizes, forms and fashions, and that's what makes us so different. The frame of the body comes in three dimensions: small, medium and large. It is important to know the dimensions of your frame, it determines your weight. Strengthening our bodies make us stronger, more able to fight diseases that attacks our bodies. We must take control and guide the body that God has entrusted to our care. The body goes through wear and tear just like anything else without proper care; however, it will not last forever. We must make the best use of our bodies by keeping healthy. What works for some people, may not work for others. The body goes through a training process and it will develop a pattern that is followed throughout life. For example, if you train your body to get up very early, you will awake every morning around the same time. You will get right up without any hesitation. The body has a natural time clock and can prompt you to arise, at a certain time. For example, whenever I want to get up at a certain time, I just program my mind the night before, and God allows me to wake-up at that specific time.

The body is so unique and so well put together that it is designed to heal itself. If we would allow the natural healing process to take place, the body would restore everything back to normal over time. There are certain things that the body needs in order to fight against the diseases that plague our bodies. We need iron, protein, magnesium, potassium, fiber and zinc. These items are essential to promote wellness for our earthly bodies; whereas, our heavenly bodies won't need any of these items. Mother Nature has designed fruits and vegetables to supply all these items above which the body needs to survive. I will elaborate on them some more in another section of the book.

First, we must take control of our bodies by learning to do those things that make us healthy. Eating the right foods, drinking plenty of water, getting enough sleep, exercising, and resting are designed so that the human body may maintain good health. The body needs wholesome food to survive and not food substitutes. These products may sound good, but there is no substitute for the real food. Although thousands of diets plans are on the market, you should use good judgment when it comes to dieting. The body needs a nutritious and well-balanced meal every day to be healthy. There is no substitute for a wholesome meal, because the body was designed to eat solid food. People consume stuff like healthy shakes, and liquid meals which are supposed to have all the vitamins and nutrition that the body needs to survive. Misuse of these products and a lack of care with these food items can do the body more harm than good.

I realize that there are some elderly people who have

poor appetites and do not desire to eat a wholesome meal every day. Some doctors recommend that they consume a type of food substitute, to provide nutrition for the body. If you are a healthy person, you do not need a substitute for food. You should eat a well-balanced and a healthy meal, at least three times a day, along with healthy snacks three or four times daily. We should be very careful about a lot of the artificial, man-made, food stuffs, which are not natural. The word artificial means not natural and is the work of human beings, not God. Anything that man has tampered with will have some type of flaws.

I recommend that you detox your body, at least four times a year, for good internal Health. My suggestion is to do it for the months of January, April, July, October, and whatever week works best for you. The first three days, you eat fruits, vegetables, and drink plenty of water, at least 8 glasses per day. After three days, you may consider a total fast (no food, just water) for one day then return to your regular meals. Many of us are walking around with toxic bodies. Detox is a form of cleaning your system and ridding the body of impurities. The older generation called it purging the body, and they used some type of laxative to detox twice each year. They did it at the beginning of spring to cover the spring and summer months, and again at the beginning of fall to cover the fall and winter months.

I can remember the awful taste of the Black Draught and Castor Oil, but they took care of our health needs. Most of our ancestors had very little education, but they had wisdom and knowledge on how to take care of their bodies. There was very little sickness and they made very few trips to the doctor's office if any at all. The only time I can remember anyone going to a doctor was when someone got hurt and needed stitches. Fruits, vegetables, and water are necessary for the body to function properly. We need to eat some type of green, leafy, vegetable every day, which helps to regulate the body function.

Secondly, the body needs plenty of water, in order to

function properly. It is pretty much like your automobile which cannot operate without gasoline. Neither does the body function well without water. So many things can happen to the body when it does not get the proper amount of water. There are such things as dehydration, urinary tract infection, and kidney disease. The body should be kept hydrated; however, it is important to drink before becoming thirsty to prevent dehydration. Lack of water can cause the body to become pale and wrinkled. Water rejuvenates the body and causes you to look younger. It gives the body radiance and glow. Water will energize the body and generate the energy that our bodies need in order to be productive. Water works miracles for the body. Not only does the body need water, but most living things need water in order to survive. Take for instance your plants, if they don't get the necessary water, they will die. Our bodies are no different. Water promotes life for our bodies. Some of our health issues stem from a lack of water.

I can remember when I hardly drank any water at all. Also, I remember some of the problems that I had, because of lack of water in my body. My lips stayed chapped, and not to mention the urinary tract infections that I encountered. I did not substitute any other beverages for water; some days, I was not drinking anything at all. There is no substitution for water---although some people try to substitute other beverages for water. I have seen people consume many type of beverages trying to quench their thirst, but it does not work. Until they consumed the water that the body needed, their thirst was not satisfied.

What really helped me to do better with my water intake was when I began to educate myself on my health issues. I learned that I could lose my kidneys if I did not drink enough water. That was an eye opener for me, because I did not want to end up having to go on dialysis in order to live. I started drinking more water and I continue to drink water daily. The first thing I reach for in the morning, when I get ready to sit and read, is water. I learned from that ordeal and I took control of my health issues. Even though I was not drinking water or any other beverages, the fact that I love watermelon could have saved me from major health issues. During the summer months, I have always eaten lot of watermelons. I still eat watermelon, but I also drink the water that my body needs. There are other items, such as fruit juices (100%, no sugar added, not from concentrate) that can help with the proper amount of liquid intake, but can never replace water. Now, I want to help other people to get a grip on their health issues. This is exactly what God wants us to do. He wants us to share good ideas with other people, to help them make the transitional.

Thirdly, the body needs sleep, to reproduce and regenerate substances for the next day or night. The body goes through a process during the time that the body is sleeping. There are certain organs that are working while the body is sleeping. Sleep is very important for the body function. A lack of sleep can cause the body to develop certain diseases and health issues. As one expert from Living Healthy explains, "Lack of sleep can cause heart disease. Research shows that sleep is good for your health, and especially for your heart." Sleep helps to boost your energy levels, promotes the ability to concentrate, and prevents the body from becoming moody. It is important to sleep without any noise, such as the radio and TV because the brain will pick up every sound. This will cause the body not get the proper sleep that it needs to function. Sometimes when you see people who are sluggish, and they went to bed early, but they did not get a good night's sleep, it's because of the noise.

Some people feel in order to fall asleep there must be some form of noise. All this is habit forming, which causes the body to become dependent upon noise in order to be able to sleep. All these things are a distraction that the body does not need. The body needs a period of silence to reboot itself, and give the brain a break after your daily tasks. We should not give anything that much power over our mind and body. We should be able to sleep in peace without any distractions, so that the body can relax. What we should do in this situation is break the cycle. Sometimes, reading the Bible can be a good source to help us fall asleep.

Next, the body needs exercise to generate energy and increase the heart rate. Some form of exercise is what keeps the body mobile. There must be some type of movement each day, in order for the body to function well. Exercise can eliminate health issues and keep us physically fit for daily chores. We must find time in our busy schedules to exercise. We must not allow laziness to cause us to develop poor health. Anything that sits up will rust-out and become unmovable. Our bodies are no different. If we don't move, we will become stiff, unable to and move freely. We must keep our limbs and muscles moving, in order to be flexible which keeps the limbs and joints healthy. We should do more standing, and less sitting. Exercise is one way to enhance mobility.

Many people lose control of bodily functions because there is not enough mobility during their daily tasks. This is the area where so many people fall short. We cannot leave the bed and go to the chair to sit all day and do nothing. For the elderly people, if we can get 9 to 15 minutes, and others 15 to 30 minutes of exercise daily, it will do wonders for our body. It does not have to be anything extreme, but anything that you feel comfortable doing to get the heart rate up. Please, do something in order to help yourself to maintain good health.

Testimony:

Dr. Kenneth T. Whalum, Jr., Pastor of The New Olivet Worship Center (The preeminent church for the teaching of true worship) in Memphis, TN., is a firm believer in exercising. He exercises, "5 days per week; 2 hours per day, consisting of a 4-mile uphill power walk and moderate weight lifting. In the words of my physician", "I'm in perfect health." (www.olivetbc.com) Dr. Whalum shows how exercising regularly will help you to maintain your weight and good health.

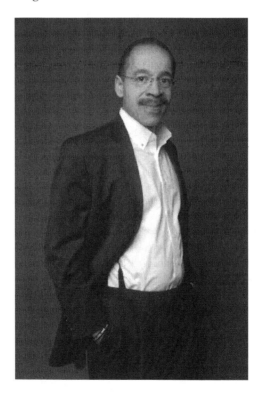

Exercise can be linked to the longevity of the Biblical characters in the Bible, because they walked for miles. Walking was their form of transportation. Even Jesus walked for miles, going from city to city to carry out His mission. This lets us know just how important exercise is for our health. I am quite sure that Christ could have had a donkey to carry Him to the different locations, but He chose to walk. I have heard of people with poor circulation, and that is likely because they did not move enough throughout the day. Walking can help poor circulation. I can truly say that walking has been the key factor for my mobility. During my younger years, I practically walked everywhere I went. I would save my bus fare and I would walk to my destination. When I attended Memphis Area Vocational School, I walked to and from class every day, except for inclement weather. This was five days a week, and it was a short distance. I have always enjoyed walking, especially early in the morning. I love to view God's creation such as, Mother Nature, smell the fresh air, cool breeze, birds singing, grass growing and flowers blooming. Spring and fall are my favorite seasons.

Finally, the body needs rest, to regroup from daily activities and gather your thoughts. The body needs peace and quiet in order to think, process and revamp in general. All of these things are important to keep the body operating smoothly and healthy. Relaxing for a few minutes will relieve tension from the body. When we rest we shut the mind down, going from operating full steam to a mood of relaxation which does wonders for the mind and body. When we do not get the proper rest the body becomes jittery and restless. After six days of labor, God rested and declared all He had made to be very good. God gives us an example to follow of how many days we should work and when to rest from our labor. The Scripture states, *"And on the seventh day God ended His work which He had made; and He rested on the seventh day from all His work which He had made"* (Genesis 2:2). Here, God demonstrates that rest is important for the body. Most Christians use Sunday as their day of rest and a day to serve God. During our day of rest, we can focus our mind and turn our attention to Godly things. We should look forward to our day of rest with the Lord, to worship and praise Him, for He is worthy of all that we have to offer Him.

When we present our whole body back to God as a living sacrifice, we acknowledge that our bodies are the Temple of Christ which does not allow us to do any and everything we desire. Therefore, with discipline, we can do as He commands. Paul says, *"I beseech you therefore, brethren, by the mercies of God, that ye present your bodies a* living *sacrifice, holy, acceptable unto God, which is your reasonable service"* (Romans 12:1). When we present our body before the Lord, we can live a God kind of life for His service. The priest no longer has to kill animals for a sacrifice for our sin and health. Jesus provided a permanent sacrifice for our sins and diseases when He went to the cross. We must begin daily laying aside our own desires to follow Him. We must put all of our trust and resources at the disposal of our Lord and Savior Jesus Christ. It's not about us and our wants but all about Jesus Christ who paid the greatest sacrifice for all man-kind. We must realize that we are not our own, because we have been bought with a price by Jesus' sacrificial act of kindness toward us. Our body belongs to God and we do not have any right to do what we want with it. We were on death row until God sent His Son to rescue us from our sins; therefore, we owe Jesus a lot when think about what He did for us.

Jesus' sacrifice should cause us to do what His disciples did. Even though Jesus had not yet been to the cross, they were willing to give up all to follow Him. He traveled throughout the land healing the sick and giving sight to blind.

CHAPTER TEN:
WHY IS TIME SO IMPORTANT?

We should spend our time wisely on things that are important; if you don't spend it wisely you'll wake-up one day and the time will be gone. In order to spend our time wisely, we must focus more on Godly things. It is so easy to get caught up in things that are worthless. Sometimes, there is just too much time spent on watching TV, lounging around, eating, and the list goes on. There is nothing wrong with these things, but the time we spend on any of them should be limited. We should spend more time focusing on more Godly and positive things. God does not mind us doing other things, but He wants us to be mindful of the time we are spending on worldly things; especially those things where God gets no glory. The Scripture says, *"See then that ye walk circumspectly, not as fools, but a wise, redeeming the time, because the days are evil"* (Ephesians 5:15). God is concerned about how we spend our time. We should also be concerned about how we spend our time, because time does not wait for us to make-up our mind to do something. It will continue to move forward whether we have used it wisely or wasted it.

Time is very precious and we should make the best out of it. We have a limited amount of time here on earth to do whatever God has destined us to do.

When I think about all the time I wasted during most of my life time, I could have done much more than what I have done. Even though I have done lots of positive things, but I know I could have done more in this frame of time. I look back at the lapse of time between my Bachelor's degree and me sitting for the CPA Exam. I graduated with my BA in May, 1989, and I did not sit for the CPA Exam until November, 1994, five years later. Then, I went back to school March, 2005, and received my Masters' degree August, 2007. There is a lot of time between these events. I look at that time and these events and I wonder if I could have done something more important with my time. I was busy doing something, but was it important? From the time I received my BA degree and the time I went back to get my Masters, is a total of fifteen years and ten months. I could have had a PhD within that length of time. Now, I was not just sitting around twiddling my thumbs. I did study and sit for the CPA Exam twice, in November, 1994 and in May 1995. I was not successful either time.

My thoughts, after the CPA ordeal, were maybe if I had taken the exam right after I received my Bachelor's degree, I may have passed the exam. Since I didn't go that route, I will never know what would have happened, if I had. One thing I do know is that I cannot correct the past, but I can change the future. One of my dreams was to become a CPA. I didn't give up on the dream, but after two attempts and not being successful either time, I decided to do something different. I am very good in the accounting area--- though I am not licensed. When I say I decided to do something different, my focus changed from numbers, to focusing on people's health on how I can make a difference in someone's life. I feel in my spirit this is what God wants me to do. Sometimes, we can have many dreams and goals, but the question becomes, do they line up with God's will for our lives? We can spend many years doing what pleases us, but not necessarily what pleases God, and what He has in mind for our destiny. When you are unsure, you can always consult with God about what He would have you do. When your will aligns with His will for your life, you will be able push your way through the obstacles that lie ahead. An obstacle can be anything or anyone that hinders you from going forward with your assignment.

The comfort of knowing God through His Word helps us to push through many of life's situations. When you get that confidence that God can handle any situation, you develop that inner peace that cannot be altered by anyone or anything that happens in your life. When you let God know that you are totally depending on Him, He comes in like a flood---He begins to work out some situations that had been denied to you. You may have been told that it cannot be done because you have messed up in the past. God comes in and says these are my children; let them have whatever they require, and I will pick up the tab. When God picks up your tab, this lets you know that you are in good standing with Him. When you get to know God through His Word, you know that He does not withhold any good thing from His children; He is a good Father who takes care of His children. When we fail to trust God, we get ourselves all stressed out and bent out of shape, over "stuff" small and big. If we could just learn to trust God for the things He has promised us, we would never be stressed out or worry about anything. When you really get to know God through His Word, you will develop a sense of peace that you cannot explain. Apply the Word of God to your everyday life. I have learned that life is so much easier when I live according to His Word. Life without the Word of God is as an empty tomb; there's no substance within.

We make God happy, by looking out for our brothers

and sisters, helping them to find their way through difficult situations. God wants us to love one another and to do right by one another. The Scripture says, *"A new commandment I give unto you, that ye love one another; as I have loved you, that ye also love one another"* (John 13:34). As Jesus is an example of God's love, we should be an example of Jesus' love to others. Showing love helps us, as believers, to stay strong in a world that is full of hatred. As a believer, I am showing love through this book, how my brothers and sisters can benefit by taking the necessary steps to eat right and to keep our temple holy, for Christ.

CHAPTER ELEVEN:
LEARNING HOW TO PREPARE
HEALTHY MEALS

The key to healthy eating is learning the techniques of preparing and seasoning food properly. There is a right and wrong way to do anything and food is no different from anything else. Many people seem to believe that if they prepare food with multiple seasonings it will make the food taste better, but that is so far from the truth, especially if those seasonings contain sodium. What usually happens is that the food is over seasoned with salt. Food will taste better and is better for the body, if you keep it simple by using a small amount of seasonings. For example, you should use one seasoning that contain sodium (seasoning salt, lemon pepper, garlic/onion salt or plain salt), and the others should have no sodium (onion/garlic powder, fennel seeds, celery seeds, Italian/poultry seasoning, sage, rosemary, oregano leaves, cumin, parsley, turmeric). The exception to this rule is, if you are an experienced cook, you can use more than one seasoning with sodium, but it should be a small amount of each.

I have seen many good vegetables turned into something unrecognizable, not to mention the taste. For example, greens when cooked with lot of onions, become overwhelmed with onion, they no longer have their natural flavor. It is a technique to prepare and to season food properly. It takes practice and patience which can be done without difficulty. There is an old saying, "practice makes perfect." Anything that is done for a while, will become natural and habitual, cooking is no different. Don't give up after the first try, continue to strive for perfection and provide healthy, sumptuous meals for your family.

When cooking for other people and large groups, as cooks we should consider all health issues, and risks of the people. We should bear some responsibility for those people trusting us to prepare their meals. Let me speak for myself as a cook, "I have a responsibility to look out for and take care of the people I cater for. We can eat ourselves back to good health by changing the way food is cooked and consumed. The proper way to season food is to start with a small amount of seasoning and as the food is almost done: you can do the taste test. The taste test helps to determine whether you should add more seasoning. Starting with a small amount of seasoning allows you to add more if needed. But you can't take it out, once it has been over seasoned. You can gradually add until you get the taste that you desire. A rule of thumb, if you use the taste test, food will never be over seasoned. I realize that the taste test cannot be used on some foods such as, meats and casseroles, but you can use good judgment. The key to seasoning meats is to sprinkle both sides lightly and rub it in, before cooking.

The way to avoid using too much seasoning together with sodium, is to read the label to determine what each contains and how much. As cooks, we must pay attention to the labels on these products to see what they contain before adding them to our food. Most of them have salt. Since the body does not consist of cells that break down salt, too much salt is not good for the body; it causes puffiness and fluid build-up. You only need a hint of salt which is a very small amount. In other words, the little personal package you get at fast food Restaurant is enough. Too much salt, over time, may also cause congestive heart failure which is a fluid build-up around the heart.

Salt may be extremely harmful for people who already have high blood pressure, low blood pressure, diabetes, high cholesterol, and kidney disease. These people must be very careful about their sodium intake. Researchers recommend that people with these health conditions use very little salt or no salt at all. Many different types of herbs are available to season food and they contain no sodium. Mrs. Dash has a line of products that can be used for people with health conditions. Salt can be used for external healing such as, in eye drops, for a sore throat, alternatively for gargling, and as a solution for congestion. A teaspoon of salt, in a cup of warm water, can work miracles for the body. Salt is good for external purposes, but should be used sparingly for internal purposes. Salt has a positive and a negative side: it can heal you but it can also kill you depending on how it is used.

Processed foods such as bacon, ham, bologna, hot dogs, smoked sausage, and all other products that are in this category should only be eaten in moderation. Also, red meat (beef) should be eaten in moderation, because it stays in your system longer and it just rots there. Red meats can cause major health problems, just like too many sweets are not good for the body, especially foods that contain lots of sugar, such as, cakes, pies, cookies, and candy bars. These foods are less harmful when eaten in moderation, and in small portions, along with your meal. They should never be eaten alone. Mints such as peppermints are ok, and can be eaten without a meal. Even with mints, and chewing gum, you must be careful not to overdo, because of harm to your teeth and your gums.

It has been stated that Americans consume more salt, sugar, and fat than any other country. If possible, bad fats should be eliminated altogether from you diet. Avoid any meat that contains a lot of fat, such as, fat back, fat pig tails, salted pork, and ox tails, because it can cause major health problems. If you must eat meat, consider seafood, fish, chicken and turkey, as these have proven to be better for your health. Fresh pork (lean) is your "other" white meat and can be eaten, in moderation, when cooked well done. This is not something that you want to do every day. Researchers are discovering more hidden secrets about foods and beverages that we are putting in our bodies. By eating right, you will be able to avoid many health issues. There are so many good foods that you can eat, until you will not miss those that are not so good for the body.

Researchers have recently discovered that Aspartame which is found in certain beverages (diet) and artificial sweeteners are causing major problems for children and adults. Parents should remove these beverages from their children's diet. Researchers now believe that ADHD a behavioral condition found in young children may be linked to the Aspartame found in the beverages that they consume. Parents are asked to pay close attention to what their children eat and drink. Aspartame may affect young children's brains and causes them to act a certain way. Also, artificial coloring found in certain foods may cause major health problems for young children. We want to protect our children by carefully checking out the food they consume. That's why I suggest that all food be cooked from scratch, which means not from a box or can, foods such as macaroni & cheese, instant potatoes, peas, beans, corn, greens, and soup. I believe you should use fresh or frozen foods, which have no additive, whenever possible. You are better able to control, what you and your family eat, by cooking your own food at home. We live in a society where we are so busy that we don't always take time to do those things that are important for our well-being. We have to take back our lives and begin to develop well-balanced lives. What it really amounts to is a reprioritization of our lives. Maybe there are some things that we should eliminate from our daily routine that are preventing us from living a balanced life. Some younger children's attitude problems stem from the food they consume which causes them to act unruly. Children with unruly behavior may have access to much of the 'bad' food, like, candy, potato chips, and sodas. We should prepare healthy foods for our families.

You should use fresh, frozen or dry foods as much as possible, because they contain no additives. Chickpeas, lentils, beans, and peas are protein-rich super foods that also pack in fiber, antioxidants, vitamin B and iron. Eating more of these foods each day, will help you control your appetite, and reduce your daily caloric intake. Beans are a good source of natural fiber. Consider pinto, great northern, black, lima beans, and navy beans. Soup is another excellent source of good nutrition, and people who eat a bowl of soup before their lunch entrees reduce their calories intake by 20%. These good wholesome foods make you feel fuller longer, and will eliminate over eating. Fast foods do no provide the nutrition that our bodies need. We must begin to take control of our health problems by making better food choices for our bodies. Vegetables, fruits, grain, and nuts are the keys to healthy eating.

It has become public knowledge that artificial sweeteners are causing health problems. Beware of diet drinks which contain artificial sweeteners; they are not good at all. They have been a factor in many health problems, such as, strokes, high blood pressure, diabetes, cancer, heart disease, and weight gain. People have been brain washed to believe that diet drinks are healthy and good for the body. They are actually doing more harm than good. Personally, I don't drink or eat anything that is labeled diet. As we begin to take health matters more seriously, and to think about the damage we are doing to our bodies; it won't be a chore to remove some of the items from our food list, and replace them with healthy choices. God is not going to remove anything from our food list: we must take that responsibility for ourselves. One article relates to artificial sweeteners as "Sweet Poison"; that's how bad they are perceived. Do you really care about your health? For example, we all know smoking causes all types of health problems which can lead to death, but that does not stop the number of youth smokers from increasing annually. Many cop out by saying, "you have to die from something." I beg to differ---I believe in my spirit that when God says our time has ended here on earth, that is when we will die and not necessarily from any specific disease. Again, remember that life and death are in the hands of God. The Word of God says we must die, but it does not say we have to have some form of disease in order to die. Dying is a part of living, as good health is a part of life.

Chapter Twelve: Cooking Tips For A Healthy Lifestyle (Meats, Vegetables, Fruits, & Nuts)

There are steps we can take to make food better and healthier. For example, any type of fowl (chicken, duck, goose, turkey) should be soaked (brining) in cold water and salt for fifteen to thirty minutes. For example, put eight pieces of chicken in a container, and add enough water to cover the chicken, approximately 1 tablespoon of salt. This will remove the blood and impurities from the meat. All meat should be cleaned before soaking. Pork spare ribs and shoulder can be soaked overnight in vinegar and cold water for tenderness. Pork, beef, venison, and lamb should be soaked in cold water and vinegar, approximately ½ cup of vinegar to enough water to cover the meat, for fifteen to thirty minutes. This will remove the impurities and blood from the meat. The blood in meats can be contaminated which could cause many health problems. When preparing meats for other dishes, the excess fat should be drained completely, especially ground beef. Also, when you bake chicken or other fowl, and there is excess fat in the broth, drain off the broth, place broth in the refrigerator or freezer to chill. After it chills, skim the fat off the top and add the broth back to your dish. You should trim all fats from meats as possible, because lean meat is better for the body. Rice and all other pastas should be rinsed and drained to remove the excess starch, which turns to sugar when consumed. There is so much that can be done to make food healthier for your body.

Eating a combination of vegetables, fruits, and nuts can help us get back to good health and maintain good health. Try removing processed and junk foods from your family's diet, and look for major improvements in your health, weight, and appetite. Some foods you will no longer acquire a taste for. The body needs live foods; raw vegetables to get nutrients naturally, which are often lost when vegetables are cooked. A glass of red wine with dinner has been listed as good for the body. For those of us who do not drink wine except for communion, drink a glass of water with two teaspoons of apple cider vinegar, and get the same results. It also relaxes the body, and allows you to get a good night's rest. Apple cider vinegar helps you to control weight, high blood pressure, promote a healthier and youthful life. Bragg Organic Apple Cider Vinegar has many good quality benefits, and can be used for healing, relaxing, cooking and cleaning.

The money currently spent on medications should be used to buy healthy food items, which are often more expensive than wholesome foods. I do not plan to spend any money on drugs, whether they are over-the- counter or prescription. I want to invest my money and energy on things that will yield a greater return on my investments. The body benefits from the consumption of vegetables, fruits, melons, beans, nuts and berries. If we give the body what it needs, we will not have to worry about most common health issues. I am living proof if you give the body what it needs to survive, you can feel good every day, without putting any drugs in your system. And that is what good health is all about, feeling good and having lots of energy. We have all seen the effects that long-term use of medications can have on the body.

You should be careful of your intake of foods that contain Trans Fats which cause heart disease and blocks blood flow in the arteries. Food that contains 'bad' fat should only be eaten in moderation, and not every day. Food such as fatback, (fat) pigtails, (fat) pig feet, chitterlings, (fat) ox tails, skins and other fried foods contain high levels of trans-fats. When eating pork chops, steaks and ribs, the leaner these meats are the better for the body. The excess fat should be trimmed off, before cooking; and only eaten in moderation. The Scripture says, *"It shall a perpetual statute for your generation throughout all your dwellings, that ye eat neither fat nor blood"* (Leviticus 3:17). God gave Moses and Aaron specific instructions concerning the meat the Israelites ate.

There are certain oils that are good for our bodies, and may be used internally and externally. They are as follows: coconut, flax seed, grape seed, hemp, olive, and peppermint. For years, coconut oil was labeled as bad fat for its high saturated-fat content. Now, it is the most popular oil on the market and considered one of the healthiest fats around. It is known for its many creative uses. The uses range from nutrition & cooking, body care, general health, and household. According to Sheila Mulrooney Eldred, "Meanwhile, recent research has also revealed that saturated fat found in coconuts --- lauric acid --- is a medium-chain triglyceride (MCT), a type of fat particularly coveted for its health and fitness benefits" (ExperienceLife.com). The olive oil is known for its many uses: it can be used for healing, facial cleanser, moisturizer, lubricant, cooking, as a salad dressing, and much more. Peppermint oil is very popular; it can be used to clear congestion and promote healing for the stomach. Two drops in a half cup of warm water daily; will work miracles for your stomach. The other oils mentioned above, have special uses, and are good for your body too.

When I was growing up, the processed meats were very good, and they were made from all natural meat, with very little fat, and no additives. They were very tasty. The luncheon meats that we buy today have many additives, made from meat by-products and they are not good for human consumption. Also, one of America's favorite snack, buttered, microwave popcorn, is not good for you. It has chemicals that can affect your lungs. Instead, air pop natural popcorn, or put natural popcorn in a brown paper bag and pop in the microwave for 2 1/2 to 3 minutes. This will eliminate all of the additives, and allow you to enjoy a favorite snack. If you decide to buy microwave popcorn, you should buy the plain microwave popcorn, without MSG or butter added. I buy the natural popcorn; put it in a small pot, with a small amount of butter (1/2 teaspoon), cover and pop. God gave man much knowledge, but man has abused and misused it for his own satisfaction. It can't be all about the mighty DOLLAR and not the safety of the consumer.

I have heard people speak about how people back in the day ate and they did not have the health problems that people experience today. Well, we must remember that most of those people worked from sun up until sun down. They were very active; therefore, they built a natural security system, to protect their bodies from many common diseases. From their hard labor, they were physically fit for their journey. Also, for people who are doing some type of physical labor or extensive exercising, they are able to control their weight and maintain a healthier lifestyle. But, what do most of our activities consist of? Sitting indoors; in office luxury, using our minds and not our bodies. There is nothing wrong with working smart, but we also must eat smart. We should not allow ourselves to become a slave to food. When our working conditions change, we should change our eating habits, to reflect our work. Once we upgrade our thinking, we can focus on the present. If you don't think there is a health crisis in our nation, just check out the hospital emergency waiting rooms.

There are people waiting to check in, as other people are waiting to check out of the hospital. Patients wait in the emergency room until a room becomes available on a floor, and other patients are released from rooms in these same areas. Hospitals all over the country experience staff shortage, unable to accommodate the overflow of patients. Staff work in these capacities are often stressed and over worked. You don't have to be one of these people, if you take control of your health, eat right, and make good choices, regarding your health. Many health problems can be traced to the food we eat. Too many bad choices of food are being consumed.

There are some foods (potato chips, candy, pastries, and sodas) that should be removed from the grocery list so that we don't bring them into our home. For example, junk foods and processed foods have become a major influence in our society. If we replace these foods with fruits and nuts, our children can reach for fruits or nuts, instead of a bag of chips or candy. Next, the intake of soda should be replaced with water or 100% natural juice. According to the Experience Life Magazine, "A 12-ounce can of soda delivers 40 grams of sugar, approximately 10 teaspoons of sugar, more than the American Heart Association's daily recommendation of 6 teaspoons per day for women, and nine teaspoons for men" (April, 2014, P. 11) The diet sodas which contain artificial sweeteners are even worse than regular sodas. They can cause excessive weight gain and contribute to other health problems. Sodas also contain lots of sodium. One can of Coke contains 45mg of sodium (salt) which is approximately 11 teaspoons of salt.

The citric acid found in sodas is also bad for your teeth. It can cause your teeth to look brown which comes from too many carbonated sodas. Recently, the size of the can of Coke has increased to a 16-ounce can which is even more sugar and sodium. This was not a grand idea to increase the size of the soda. The entire family has to be protective of their good health; remove these harmful foods and beverages from their diets especially for children, who will suffer the most. As individuals, we can begin to transition, and change our life style, for the better. Start now, in order to change the next generation.

There are so many hidden ingredients in our food that can wipe us out. Controlling sugar, salt, and fat intake can prevent major health problems. If you eat these items in low quantity, you can prevent many of the health issues known to be influenced by, sugar, salt and fats. I have seen people sit down to eat, and before they take the first bite of food; they start sprinkling salt on their food. This is a bad habit, because raw salt is worse than salt that is cooked in the food. When salt is cooked in the food, it dissolves evenly throughout the cooking process which makes it less harmful and more easily digested than raw salt.

Parents have a big responsibility to help their children make better healthy choices, especially when selecting food items at school. If children are trained to eat healthy, they will begin to make healthy choices throughout their lives. This teaching must begin in the home. Parents, as we educate our children about food choices and teach them that having a piece of fruit or a salad, instead of a bag of chip or French fries is a better food choice. Let them know why fruit and salad over chips and French fries is better for their bodies. They must be told about unhealthy foods and why these food choices can lead to ill health in the future. Some parents may believe that because children are growing, they can eat anything, without ill effects. That is so far from the truth. Growing children can have the same diseases as older people. The entire family must work together for a common cause.

It is important to get children involved in making healthy decisions while they are young, so that they can grow up making good health choices in life. This bad habit cycle can be broken so our children do not carry them over into the next generation. Generational curses have to stop somewhere. It's just like anything else that is not of God. It's not in God's will that anyone should perish; God specializes in health, but not disease. As Christians, turning our health around allows us to better serve God, so that He gets the Glory. We are being disobedient when we don't take care of our health. God gets no glory when we are sick and unable to serve. We were created to serve God. If we are ill then God's Kingdom work is being short changed by our illness.

Here, I will provide a list of healthy tips of vegetables, fruits, berries, and nuts that can correct many of your health problems, and help you get back to good health. If you include these vegetables, fruits, berries, and nuts in your daily eating, they will eliminate many of your health issues. God has created healing foods for every condition. By eating yourself back to good health, you do not have to worry about the side effects of medications. You will begin to feel better every day by doing things naturally. You don't have to worry about dieting you just need to eat a healthy meal. I know there are times when your body is under attack by Satan, and there is a need for a temporary fix, to get some relief from pain. That's why it's so important to use the prevention method, before problems arise. Mother Nature has the best healing power provided by God, for His people.

Let's look at some of the prevention foods for the body's health issues. All types of cancer can be prevented by eating a combination of these fruits and vegetables: apples, grapefruits, strawberries and raspberries, which contain ellagic acid and antioxidants that destroys cancer cells throughout the body. The vegetables are carrots, pumpkins, sweet potatoes, and red peppers which have beta-carotene. Cauliflower, broccoli, and raw cabbage also fight against cancer. The vegetables that contain beta-carotene also prevent heart diseases and strokes. The beta-carotene should come from food and not from supplements. Cherries are a cure for gout. Apricots can enhance your love life. Celery, purple potatoes, and fresh garlic can lower blood pressure. High cholesterol can be lower by eating oatmeal, cinnamon, ginger, walnuts, almonds, flaxseed, pears, oranges and avocados. Birth defects, heart disease, cancer, and high blood pressure can be eliminated by eating watermelons which contain vitamin A. A cut onion can be used on bugs bite such as, bees and mosquitoes to stop the stinging and itching. It has anti-inflammatory power which also helps asthma suffer to breathe freely. Bananas, oranges, sweet potatoes, carrots, beans, cantaloupes, and beets are high in potassium. Beets and turnip greens also build iron poor blood. By stocking up on vegetables, fruits, berries, and nuts, you can eliminate medications. I am speaking from personal experience and information gathered from researching.

Researchers have discovered that Mother Nature has the best medicine and cure for the body. I was able to get my husband, Edward to incorporate more fruits in his diet. He took a love for the red pear; he eats it daily. Lately, he has been eating apples and bananas. He tells me how much better he feels, since he started eating more fruits. He has access to all types of fruits, but chooses to eat pears, apples, and bananas. I keep plenty of fruits; because they are part my daily meal. We must get back to the basis by realizing that good health comes from the farm and not the pharmacy. Vitamins are not a necessity when you eat fruits, vegetables, nuts, beans and berries daily. You must remember that vitamins are supplements and they cannot replace a well-balanced meal. You can be assured that pills, as small as they are, cannot substitute for a well-balanced meal. They can aid people who do not eat healthy, but they alone cannot implement good health.

Chapter Thirteen: Losing Weight The Natural Way

The first step when deciding to lose weight is to minister to you. Why do you want to lose weight? How do you plan to lose weight? What do you expect to achieve from losing the weight? What plan should you have in place to help you maintain your weight? These are questions to be asked of yourself so that you can program your mind and carry out your plan. When you take these steps your mind will begin to work with your body. If the mind does not know what the body is planning to do, it becomes a conflict of interest because the mind and body are not working together. The next thing to do is to voice your weight lost goal to someone who will support your ideas and help you to meet your goal. More than likely, by following these simple steps, you will lose the weight and keep it off. What happens to most people who gain the weight back is that they had no plans as to how they would maintain their weight loss.

There is always a wrong and right way to do anything. You should never use the words "dieting" or "diet" because you will lose the weight, and nine times out of ten you gain it all back and more. The words you should use are "change eating habits" or "lifestyle". By taking this approach, you are more likely to lose weight and keep the weight off. Also, you must set a goal for losing weight that considers how much weight you plan to lose and the amount of time needed to lose the weight. Your plans should be written down so that you will be able to refer back to your goals and track your progress. Having a support system in place is always good; to have someone who can share in your progress. You should begin to make changes to your lifestyle by changing the way you eat such as how, what, and when.

One big mistake that I have seen people make is eating larger meals at night and then going to bed. You can't work it off, so the food ends up turning into lots of fat. The next mistake is eating in the bedroom or lounging on the sofa and not eating in the kitchen. Each room has a purpose and is designed for certain usages. Schwartz says, "People eat what's easiest to access and what they can see" (Schwartz, Dec. 2012, Rudd Center for food policy 'on' obesity). The best food choices are made in your kitchen, where you can control the food that is available to your family. Losing weight can be a challenge, but the most effective way to lose weight is to do it the proper way.

The five most important things that will assist you with weight loss are as follows: (1) Drink plenty of water; (2) eat three well balanced meals, beginning with breakfast, eat healthy snacks in between meals each day; (3) get proper rest; (4) exercise, and (5) sleep. These steps are preventive maintenance for the body. When lacking in any of these areas, the body will begin to show signs of malfunction, such as dehydration, stress, lack of energy, and low balance. These warning signs indicate the body is not getting everything it needs to function properly. But most of the time, these warning signs are ignored. These steps are an important part of the body's metabolism. Everyone's metabolism is different. Some people have to do more and work harder in order to maintain a proper weight. Some people can do less, and get the same result. In order to maintain good health, you should consider these steps.

For instance, water is a purifier for the body, which the body needs a certain amount of each day, in order to work properly. Water eliminates and removes the waste material from the body. Water enhances body functions, hair, nail, and skin. Water also flushes the kidneys and helps them to function well, and keeps the body from becoming dehydrated. Water can be a cure for everything that ails us. It gives the body nutrients and radiance. Sometimes, we try to substitute other beverages for water. It cannot and should not be done. There's nothing that can take the place of water in your system. Water is a natural element and cost little to provide. I can remember when water was free of charge in my home town. Water is so important that God gathered it before He gathered the dry land. The Scripture says, *"And God said, let there be a firmament in the midst of the waters, and let it divide the waters from the waters. And God made the firmament, and divided the waters which were under the firmament, from the waters which were above the firmament: and it was so. And God said, let the waters under the heaven be gathered together unto one place, and let the dry land appear: and it was so"* (Genesis 1:6-7, 9). Water was created before the earth because the earth's survival depends upon water.

The body make up is 70 percent water. That's why it is so important to drink the required amount of water, which is a recommended minimum eight glasses daily. When we do not drink the proper amount, our urine is yellow in color. But when we drink the water we need each day, the urine will be clear. Water plays a major role in our health condition. There is no substitute for water. Often people try to use other beverages to quench their thirst, but they never work. Water is one of the key sources to a healthy life, and a lack of water will cause the body to become dehydrated. Some people believe that increasing their caffeine intake will help them burn more calories, which may hold true to some degree, but caffeine is a diuretic, and diuretics cause dehydration. You should drink more water and decrease your caffeine intake. There are certain organs of the body that depends on water to function properly. For example, if our kidneys do not get the proper water needed to function, the liver will pick up the slack which causes it to become over worked and lower overall productivity. The liver has its own important body functions and should not be carrying the responsibility of the kidneys. The kidneys cannot function well if they are water-deprived. When we do not drink the proper amount of water, the body begins to store and hold on to whatever water we take in.

Water can be used to curb the appetite. If you drink an 8-oz. glass of water before each meal, you will not eat as much, because water is filling. Then, if you drink an 8-oz. glass of water after each meal, you will continue to curb the appetite. You should drink an 8-oz glass of water before and after breakfast, lunch and dinner. We should have a snack in the morning, one in the afternoon and one light snack at night. Depending on your meal, snacking may not be necessary. Sometimes, water can take the place of a snack, because it makes you feel full. This will give you the amount of recommended water that you should drink each day. Another method of utilizing water is to drink two cups or one 16.9 oz. bottle of water; thirty minutes before each meal, you'll see immediate result in your weight. By losing weight, you will eliminate many health problems and issues, related to obesity. If you are having health problems, because of your weight, lose the weight and achieve the desired result.

Testimony:

Valarie lost 145 pounds, and no longer has diabetes or high blood pressure.

My lifestyle changed because I had to remember, to eat small meals more frequently. I have to set my alarm clock to remind me every two hours, so that I won't forget.

In 1994, I was diagnosed with systemic Lupus. Due to medications and eating all the wrong foods, over the years, I gained 315 pounds. In February 2013, I was diagnosed with Type II Diabetes. In July 2013, I had gastric bypass surgery. Today I've lost 145 pounds and no diabetes.

I eat small meals every two hours. This consists of a small breakfast (8:00 am); small fruit (10:00 am), Lunch (12:00 noon); small fruit or yogurt (2:00 pm) Dinner at (5:00 pm) snack at (8:00 pm). Drink water throughout the day. I don't eat beef, pork, bread, and sweets.

It is amazing how a simple lifestyle change can make all the difference for better health. During our conversation, Ms. Wright talked about how much better she feels since losing the weight. Prior to her surgery, she had limited activities outside of her home. Now, she is able to attend social functions. She is able to enjoy life again with her children. To God be the glory!

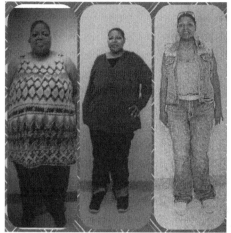

Before   After

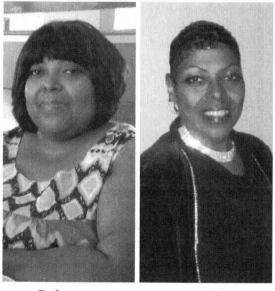

Before   After

The next thing that will help one to lose weight is maintaining good eating habits, which is essential to good health and weight loss. Especially for people who are trying to lose weight or maintain a desired weight. One cannot lose weight by eating one big meal a day, because the body will begin to store up everything you consume. The body will pick up on any irregular meal habits. The body senses that you are not going to feed it regularly, and it will hold on to anything you consume. When the body reaches this stage, you will not lose any weight. Eat regularly so that the body can get the needed daily nutrients. Eating three well balanced meals and snacks throughout the day, keeps the body from feeling hungry. When the body feels hungry, one tends to over eat. In between breakfast and lunch, lunch and dinner, one should find healthy snack foods to eat.

For example, raw veggies (carrots, broccoli, cauliflower, tomatoes, cucumbers, and celery); fruits (apples, grapes, oranges, pears, peaches, bananas, cherries and kiwifruit); berries (strawberries, raspberries, blueberries, and blackberries); and nuts (peanuts, almonds, and walnuts); are good snack foods to eat. You can't lose weight by starving yourself; you lose weight by eating more of the right foods. Do not waste your money on diet foods. Researchers have discovered that diet foods are doing more harm than good. You should invest in all natural foods.

We must learn to rest from our labor. Sometimes this means taking a few minutes from our labor to rest our bodies and to regroup. A few minutes of rest can make a world of difference in how well we function. Most importantly, we must take at least one whole day from our labor to rest. Rest is an important factor in healthy living. God ceased from His labor, after creating the universe in six days. The Scripture says, *"And on the seventh day God ended His work which He had made; and He rested on the seventh day from all His work which He made. And God blessed the seventh day, and sanctified it: because that in it He had rested from all His work which God created and made"* (Genesis 2:2-3). God sat the example for us to follow. If God rested from His labor, then most assuredly we can rest from our labor.

Exercise is the key to changing your body. If we incorporate exercise into our busy schedules, we will be on our way to a healthier lifestyle. Exercise keeps our bodies physically fit and boosts our energy levels. It also helps us to lose and maintain our weight, and build stronger bodies. If we exercise as little as nine minutes a day, and no more than thirty minutes, it will do marvelous things for the heart, especially for the older generation. Getting our heart rate up every day stimulates the heart muscle, as it pumps the blood through the body. There are many forms of exercise. For example, house cleaning, gardening, aerobics, walking, running, dancing, skating, biking, and playing ball are all good forms of exercise. By exercising, we can prevent many of our health issues and correct others.

We feel good and look better when we exercise. We should keep our bodies mobile by any means necessary. People get in their mind, when they get a certain age that they can't do certain things and life stops. Excuses will make you lazy and complacent. You can reach a point in life where you believe you can do nothing right. When you are in this negative mindset, it is hard to get yourself up and back out of there, and on the right track. The best advice is to avoid getting in a slump. Are you one of those people who never have a good day? Moaning and groaning about something every God sent day? Exercise helps keep your mind and thoughts clearer; your body will be more energized and capable of defeating illness and disease.

Finally, the body also needs sleep. In order for your organs to function properly and your body to generate the substance needed, you need rest. Not getting the proper amount of sleep can contribute to health problems and overall ill health. For the body to thrive sleep is a very important factor. Functioning well means you are getting 'good' sleep not restless sleep. Adults do not require as much sleep as children. With seven hours each night, adults will do well. Sometimes this is where I find myself falling short, when it comes to sleep. There are some nights when I get very little sleep. But I have begun to do better, because I know how important sleep is to my overall well-being and good health. If I stay up late one night, the next night I will go to bed early. The problem is that you can't make-up for lost sleep. You need to make sure you get the proper hours of sleep every night or day, if this works better for you. You should love your body inside and outside. When you are in love with your body, you'll treat it well, and you want what's best. Don't revert back to the same bad eating habits, due to stress or lack of focus, which is easy to do when something happens (usually bad) to cause us to lose control.

The most important factor to losing weight is learning how to maintain and control it after losing the weight. Most people will lose the weight and they end up gaining it back and some more. You must have a plan in place, so when you lose the weight you won't go back to that same lifestyle. If you had a goal for losing the weight, you must have one more goal for keeping the weight off. In other words, when you begin to lose the weight, you must have a strategy in place of how you are going to maintain and control your weight lost. I have seen so many people go to great extreme and sacrifice to lose a lot of weight, but they ended up putting it right back on. They reverted back to their same bad eating habits. Sometimes because something happened in their lives to cause then to lose control, for example, a state of depression, low self-esteem and not being able to focus on what things are of value. At this point, you need a whole lot of Jesus and less food.

CHAPTER FOURTEEN:
A PRODUCTIVE LIFESTYLE

In order to live a productive, healthy lifestyle, we, especially Christians, must live according to the Word of God. If we take the Word of God and apply it to our everyday lives, we can eliminate some of the problems we face each day. Jesus tells us to, *"Come unto me all ye that labor and are heavy laden; and I will give you rest."* (Matthew 11:28). Jesus tells us that we can give it all to Him and we can relax. He does not want us to get bogged down with health issues. He wants us to be free to serve Him. Our mission here, as Christians, is to serve God and make the world a better place. We can make a difference in this world by allowing people to see Christ within us. We must begin to represent Christ in all walks of life. Our goal in this life should be to exemplify Christ in everything we do and everywhere we go. For example, I was asked to help with a repast, for a friend of the family, whose mother passed away. The repast was at a club, and I had to exemplify Christ in that situation. There could have been someone who did not know Jesus. Living for Christ is a full time commitment. We must live a Christ-like life twenty-four hours a day, seven days a week.

There is so much sickness and disease in the world today. There has to be a reason for all of these dilemmas. Things just don't pop-up out of nowhere; they stem from something. Faith in God is not enough we must trust Him to do just what He said in His word. God will always come through for His people. We may fall short of our promises, but God always keeps His promises. He is God and He cannot and will not lie. Sometimes, we just need to examine ourselves and make sure we are in a right standing position with God. God never moves; therefore, if anyone moved, it was us. When we remove ourselves from the will of God, we open ourselves up to all types of problems, including health issues and mistakes. The good news is, God never moved! He may be found in His word and through the Holy Spirit.

I often wonder why there is so much sickness and disease. I can remember going to the hospital to visit a sick church member. I drove around about ten minutes trying to find somewhere to park. I just don't recall having a parking problem, at the hospital, in the past. It appears that the hospitals are over crowded with sick people, and their families visiting. Is there an epidemic of illness plaguing our community? If God has not changed, then the burden to change the condition of our society relies upon us. It is crucial to stay in the Will of God; however, God gets no pleasure or joy from our illness, financial problems, or family matters that are not going well in our lives. On the other hand, Satan gets great joy when Christians are struggling to make ends meet. The enemy will try to keep us down, but we must remember that we serve a mighty God who is all powerful. The devil is no match for Him and His Word will cause the enemy to flee from us. God will bless us if we diligently seek Him. We may have trials and tribulations, but they are only for a season. One of Satan's biggest tricks is to get us to doubt the love God has for us. There are reasons why God allows us to go through some difficult times. Trials and tribulations that we encounter are to make us stronger and we may be a living testimony for someone else.

The life of Job is a perfect example for us to follow. The Scripture tells us that, *"So the Lord blessed the latter end of Job more than his beginning: for he had fourteen thousand sheep, and six thousand camels, and a thousand yoke of oxen and a thousand she asses"* (Job 42:12). Our situations can be used to help others grow when they are going through. We can provide comfort needed to endure and overcome life's difficult times in our lives. Paul tells us: *"Blessed be God, even the Father of our Lord Jesus Christ, the Father of mercies, and the God of all comfort; who comforts us in all our tribulation, that we may be able to comfort them which are in any trouble, by the comfort wherewith we ourselves are comforted of God"* (2 Corinthians 1:3-4). God is a great comforter; He allows us to put our cares in His hand and lean on Him, for He is with us always.

We are never alone, for the presence of God is with us and where we find peace. The Scripture tells us that God will be with us, *"Lo I am with you always, even unto the end of the world"* (Matthew 28:20). God is with us through the Holy Spirit. Each believer has access to the Holy Spirit, whom we can depend on to lead and guide us. We'll find we make better decisions and choices if the Holy Spirit orders our steps. Don't rely on your own understanding, but seek knowledge from the Holy Spirit who knows all things. Whenever I ask the Holy Spirit to reveal something to me, He is always there to assist me with everything I require. Even in the simple things, like locating something I thought I lost, the Holy Spirit brings to my attention immediately and I know exactly where to look. I don't hesitate to call upon the Holy Spirit for help. The presence and power of God dwells in all believers through the Holy Spirit. So, whatever we stand in need of, whether it's losing or controlling our weight, maintaining a balanced life, eating our way back to good health, the Holy Spirit is ever present.

God wants us to be as little children, totally leaning and depending on Him to take care of all of our needs. He wants to continue to show His affection for us as we live according to His Word. When we have that personal relationship with God, we have a direct connection with Him, through the Holy Spirit. That's why it is so important to invite the Holy Spirit to dwell within our souls. When we are in the right relationship with God, He will supply all of our needs and will give us the desires of our heart. It pays to have a personal relationship with God. I have received so many wonderful blessings from God, until sometimes I feel like a spoiled child. When I call on my Daddy, He comes to my rescue. When I don't know what to do, He's always there to assist me and direct me in the right direction. I am so happy to have someone who watches over me, looks out for me, takes care of my every need, and who does not allow anyone to take advantage of me. It feels so good to have genuine protection from a powerful God. There is no need for us to be concerned about food, shelter, clothing, and health. God has promised to take care of all our needs on earth and in heaven.

For example, God has always looked out for me when I didn't understand a lot about life. I can remember when I didn't have any food to prepare dinner for my family. I got up that morning and prepared breakfast for my family. I didn't have to be concerned about lunch, my ex-husband was at work and my children were at school. I had no idea, what I was going to do about dinner. What I know now, but didn't know then, God had already provided for dinner. There was a knock at the door, I looked out; it was Mr. and Mrs. Jones, my uncle and aunt. They came by to take me grocery shopping. I never called anyone about my situation. God sent them my way, he is my survival kit and He has everything I need to survive. When I look back over my life, I know it was Him watching over me. I am so grateful to God for doing so.

Like any loving father, He cares about the need of His children. He does not want us to seek advice from other sources. God wants us to totally put all of our trust in Him. Even when we face disappointments, we must continue to put all our trust in the Lord. He has all of the answers to our problems and He is the only one who can solve them. Most of the time, we consult with everybody except God. Even though He already knows, He still wants us to converse with Him. I am often reminded of the song, "What a friend we have in Jesus." There is a line that says, "Oh what needless pain we bear, all because we do not carry everything to Him in prayer." There is so much truth to those words, God is right there, waiting to help us with everything we need. But, we are free agents, and God allows us to make our own choices. We must come to Him freely because He is able and willing to help us in every way.

God really wants us to have the best life ever. He wants to capture our hearts and build that special relationship with us. His love for us is unconditional and indescribable; he will never break our hearts. Therefore, God wants us to return His love unconditionally. God has a plan for our future that supersedes any of our past failures. If you listen to the devil, he will make you think that everything is over for you and that you cannot begin again. The devil hates God so much that he will do anything to destroy God's people. We cannot get caught up in his mess, and we certainly do not want to be a part of his kingdom. The most important thing about past failures is that we should learn from them so that we do not repeat them in the future.

Sometimes, God allows us to go through sickness, disease, and ill health in order to develop us for the future plans He has for us to carry out and to move to the next level. He develops our character to fit His agenda. God did not allow me to be successful in the restaurant business. I have learned that God has reasons for whatever He does at the time, and that He is working it out for our good. The Scripture says, *"And we know that all things work together for our good to them that love God to them who are the called according to His purpose"* (Roman 8:28). God works out all things---not just isolated incidents---for our good. This does not means that everything that happens to us is good, because evil is prevalent in our fallen world. It means that God is able to turn it around, for our good. Even though, at the moment, I don't understand why some things turn out the way they do, but I go to God in prayer, and He helps me to understand better.

We should keep in mind that God's way is always better, and will always yield the most benefits for our life. I realize in order to live a healthy and victorious life, I must allow God to take control of my life and take care of my needs. God already knows what I need before I even ask Him. He specializes in fulfilling the necessities of life for His people. There are benefits to being connected to the right source, God the Father, God the Son, and God the Holy Spirit. When we are not connected to the right source, the devil comes in like a flood and sweeps us away. If we are safe in the arms of God, he can't touch us unless God allows him to do so, and God gets the glory. Satan will use anything possible, to destroy God's kingdom. Satan hates God and His people; he will do anything in his power to destroy the people of God. When God gives us something of value, good health, peace and happiness, the enemy will try to take it away.

God can reverse anything that Satan allows because God is all power. It is true that God is always in control in every situation, so, we have no reason to be intimidated by Satan's limited power on earth. For example, when Satan destroys something, God can restore it. When Satan brings sickness, God sends healing. When Satan causes sadness, God generates happiness. When Satan causes weakness, God releases strength, for the joy of the Lord is our strength. Satan "arms are too short" and are no match for

God. God takes our shattered lives and mends them back together. Unlike humpty dumpty, "all of the king's men and king's horses could not put humpty back together again." God is able to take your worse situation, death, disease, sickness, and turn it into something beautiful. Satan cannot do any more than what God allows him to do. Job's situation is an excellent example: God allowed Satan to touch job's body but he could not touch his soul.

God is such a loving Father and that is His reason for wanting to shield us from destruction. He really wants to bless us and not harm us. He wants His people to be prosperous in everything. We block our blessings when we don't follow the instructions that God has given us. We bring sorrow and pain when we disobey God's instructions and His commands. A right relationship with God, will give us hope for a brighter future. The Scripture says, *"For I know the thoughts that I think toward you, says the Lord, thoughts of peace, and not evil, to give you an expected end"* (Jeremiah 29:11 KJV). God is great and He encourages His people through His word to move toward a better life. It does not mean that we will be spared suffering, pain, or hardship but that God will see us through all of our problems. He will not forget His people and He will honor their every need according to His Word.

You must be aware of every situation including your health. While it may be a struggle, the whole armor of Christ is going to get you through every struggle. We will not give up and we will not give in, for failure is not of God. You must remember my brothers and my sisters; we are in this fight for the win. There are going to be some pitfalls along the way but be encouraged, you will overcome each of them. God has not equipped you to be hopeless, but to be powerful, to take back any territory that enemy has stolen, including your health, peace, and joy.

CONCLUSION: USING YOUR POWER AND STRENGTH

This book is based on Biblical Principles, which is from God's perspective. The Bible, my personal experience, and research from other reliable sources were used to write this book. You gain power and strength through the Word of God. This book shows how you get everything you need by reading and studying His Word. There's so much important information in this book, and it is designed to change the world's perspective on health issues and drugs. This is not to judge or condemn, but to encourage and inform you of information for a better you. All good things are linked to our Creator. I want to show how everything is connected to the word of God. You should read with eyes of faith, belief, trust, and know whatever your situation is, it can be changed. This book is to educate people on health issues that can be corrected. It is so important for believers to become the vehicle to sustain good health, set examples, and be able to help the rest of the world with health problems.

As I conclude, my hope is, you will use the information from this book, to make the transition for a better you and your family. God has provided every tool you need to take control of your health. This book offers those tools you need from start to finish. My prayer is, after reading this book you will make it a priority to change your eating habits and lifestyle. Please, don't put it away, not to be picked up again, allow this book to become a guide for healthy living. It is up to you, to take the initial step to improve your health condition and get rid of those issues you don't need. God gives you strength to overcome obstacles, hindering and anything holding you back.

TAKE CONTROL OF YOUR HEALTH

Through much research, my task is to educate people about healthy eating, lifestyle changes, and prescription drugs. My hope is, not to lose another generation to illness and disease due to lack of knowledge. It takes a little time to educate yourself on foods that are 'good', not so good and those that are 'bad' for your health. There may be times when you need to take prescription drugs temporarily. It should not be for a life time. Before taking any medication, be sure to research and check it out for side effects. That's why I recommend you to prevent these issues from happening. In the meantime, you should be putting together a healthy meal plan to get you back to good health. I have done the leg work, you just need to apply the information to correct or prevent health issues. I just want people to become more concerned with their health.

My task was to search the Scripture for answers in regards to sicknesses and diseases, and to show you a more excellent way to handle your health issues. We find everything we need to know in the Word of God; how everything should be done. I was able to gather information to support my belief; sicknesses and diseases are not the plan that God has for believers. His plan is to, prosperous us, not harm us, and to give us a bright future.

The key is to gain knowledge through the Word of God, by reading, studying, and allowing the Holy Spirit to teach, lead, and guide us. He gives you an understanding of what you have read and studied. Just think! Do you believe that God wants His people plagued with the sicknesses and diseases we see today? No, what God wants is for His people to have life and more abundantly.

USE YOUR WEAPON

Don't allow the enemy to control your life with sickness and disease. You have the power to take back what the enemy has stolen from you. You have been equipped through the Word of God. You have been carrying your weapon, which is the Word of God, but you have not aimed at anything. You should use your weapon to kill those things which are not good for your health. Use your weapon to get rid of those things not pleasing to God and are not good for your life. Those things have been listed for you in this book. Use the example of the hunter who uses his weapon to aim and shoot. If you never aim at anything, you will never kill anything. You have the resource; give it your best shot.

My hope is, when people read this book, they realize there is a more excellent way of life. We should not fill our bodies with drugs, whether prescription or over-the-counter. Mother Nature has provided for us those things needed for our bodies in order to maintain good health. You may have lost sight on those things God intended for our lives. This book will guide you and help you get on track. We should not relate to health issues as the world sees them. As true believers, God makes it clear; we will be of the world but not a part of it. This book is designed to help people get back to the basic way of life, which is the way the Creator designed it.

APPENDIX A

Recipes are simple and easy to follow.

SUCCOTASH

3 cups corn (white/yellow) (fresh/frozen)	¾ tsp seasoned salt
1 ½ cups cut okra (fresh/frozen)	½ tsp garlic powder
2 medium diced tomatoes (red)	½ tsp onion powder
1 tbsp. canola oil	

Mix all ingredients together and heat oil in skillet. Pour mixture into hot skillet. Cook over medium heat about fifteen minutes or until tender; stirring occasionally. Taste for seasoning; add more if needed.

CHICKEN VEGETABLE SOUP

1 lb. frozen mixed vegetables	1 ½ cups corn (12 oz. fresh/frozen)
1 ½ cups cut okra (12 oz. fresh/frozen)	½ cup chopped onion (optional)
½ cup chopped celery (optional)	½ bell pepper (optional)
2 large potatoes (diced)	3 large tomatoes (diced)

Combine mix vegetables, corn, okra, onion, celery, bell pepper, potatoes, diced tomatoes and salt in pot with four cups of water. Cook about 15 minutes or until tender. Add cooked chicken to soup and continue to cook for five minutes. Tomatoes should be boiled about two minutes to remove the skin, dice and add to soup. Taste for seasoning and season to your taste. Other spices may be used (Fennel Seed, Oregano, Rosemary, Garlic Powder & Onion Powder)

SALISBURY STEAK

1 lb. ground turkey	¾ tsp Weber Gourmet Burger seasoning
1 tsp seasoned salt	¾ tsp garlic powder
1 tsp onion powder	1 egg
½ cup flour	¼ onion, sliced thin
4 tbsp. oil	

Mix all ingredients except for flour and onion. Shape meat into five steaks. Place the ½ cup of flour in a shadow pan. Battle the steaks on each side with flour and remaining flour maybe used for gravy. Place three tbsp. of oil in skillet and heat over medium heat until hot. Place the steak in hot skillet and brown on each side. Put browned steaks to the side. Use the same skillet to brown flour and onion for gravy. Put 1 Tbsp. oil in skillet; add four tbsp. of flour stir until slightly brown; add onion and continue to brown flour and onion. Put steaks back in skillet. Add 2 1/2 cups of water and bring to a boil. Reduce heat and simmer until gravy thickens to desired consistency.

CHICKEN, RICE & BROCCOLI CASSEROLE

4 ½ cups cooked rice (parboiled)	4 cups cut broccoli, cooked
4 cups cubed chicken, cooked	1 26 oz. can Cream of Chicken Soup (low sodium)
8 oz. shredded Cheddar cheese	

Preheat oven to 375. Combine the first four ingredients. Mix well and pour into 13x9 or 11 x 8 ½ pan. Top with cheese, and bake for 35 minutes, or until slightly brown.

TOSSED COMBINATION VEGETABLE/FRUIT SALAD

1 16 oz. Mixed Salad Greens	1 pint cherry Tomatoes or 4 medium vine (sliced)
1 lg cucumber	½ lb. strawberries (sliced)
1 apple, diced	½ lb. grapes
1 cup shredded carrots	½ purple cabbage, shredded
1 ½ cups cut broccoli	1 cup cut celery
1 10 oz. bag baby spinach	3 eggs (sliced)
2 cups diced cooked chicken	

Wash, combine and toss all fruits and vegetables. Use Italian lite salad dressing or apple cider vinegar and olive oil.

APPENDIX B

TIPS AND GUIDANCE

I. What you should do before and during doctor visits.
1. Pray before going to the doctors.
2. Let your doctor know that you are a believer.
3. Ask questions concerning your health.
4. Let him or her know your opinion about taking medication.
5. Check all prescription drugs before consuming for side effects.
6. Take control of your health by changing lifestyle through food and exercising.
7. Mother Nature has provided for us everything we need.

II. What you should do when there is a serious illness.
1. It's wise to get a second opinion.
2. Mostly, seeking guidance through the

Holy Spirit.
3. Don't be afraid when you receive unpleasant news; God has not given us the spirit of fear.
4. Remember, God is with you; He will never leave you nor forsake you.
5. Remember, there is nothing too hard for God to fix.
6. Remember, your healing comes through God and not man.
7. Mount up with wings as an eagle and soar to your healing
III. Don't be misguided by the enemy (Satan).
1. Let Satan know who you are taking your instructions from.
2. Never give up on God, He has your back.
3. Remember, God is all power and Satan's power is limited.
4. Pray, believe, trust, and watch God work it out.
5. Remember, life and death is in the hands of God.
6. Remember, God is the giver of life and He gives it abundantly.
7. Stay motivated and excited about life.
IV. Develop good eating habits
1. Eat plenty vegetables, fruits, and nuts daily.
2. Drink lots of water, natural juice, and (almond, rice, and coconut) milk.
3. Avoid sugar, salt, and fat as much as possible; use sparingly.
4. Incorporate healthy fat in your diet (avocado, coconut, hemp oil).
5. Avoid processed foods as much as possible.

6. Never become addicted to food; control your intake.

7. Remember, Mother Nature has provided everything you need.

V. Keep your body mobile

1. Exercise at least three times a week.

2. Don't sit too long; move as frequently as possible.

3. Stay active doing something; it's good for the mind and body.

4. Anything that sits up over time will rust and become unmovable.

5. Meditating on the Word of God is good exercise for the mind.

6. Become proactive and not reactive.

7. Take care of your body when you are young; it will serve you well.

APPENDIX C: HEALTHY TIPS

Pistachio: healthy nuts good for snack.

Bananas: cure for stress or anxiety 30% B6 vitamin.

Yogurt: cure for constipation or gas.

Raisins: cure for high blood pressure; they are high in potassium.

Apricots: preventing kidney stones; also high in potassium.

Tuna: cure for a bad mood; so eat your way to happiness.

Ginger tea: cure for nausea; ¼ teaspoon of ginger powdered, ½ to 1 Teaspoon of minced ginger root or a cup of ginger tea can ease nausea and motion sickness during pregnancy.

Basil: cure for tummy troubles, studies suggest that eugenol; a compound in basil, can keep your gut safe from pain, nausea, cramping, or diarrhea by killing off bacteria such as, salmonella and listeria, according to Mildred Mattbeldt-Beman, MD, use minced or fresh basil in sauces or salad.

Pear: cure for high cholesterol: It has 5g of fiber, much of it in the form of pectin, helps flush out bad cholesterol.

Buckwheat honey: cure for coughing; 2 teaspoons of dark brown honey; where honey's antioxidants and antiviral

Cabbage: cure for ulcers, provides 3g of fiber and vitamin C: It has been found that the powerful compound in cabbage help control the Helicobacter pylori bacteria that causes gastric peptic ulcers.

Turkey: cure for sleepless nights; 3 ounces of turkey has nearly all the tryptophan (an essential amino acid that helps the body produce a serotonin and melatonin harmony) that regulates sleep you need a day. According to La Puma studies show that people who suffer from Insomnia is deficient in tryptophan.

Figs: cure for Hemorrhoids. The 3g of fiber in four dried figs help create, soft stool. It keeps hemorrhoids from returning. Figs also provide about 5% of daily potassium and 10% manganese.

Orange juice: for fatigue 4 ounce glass is a perfect pick me up, says Gerbstadt. The vitamin C has the ability to combat oxidative stress, may also provide energy and plays a key role in metabolizing iron.

Garlic: cure for yeast infection. Garlic contains essential oils that can inhibit the growth of candida albicans fungus, the culprit in the pain, itch, and vaginal discharge of yeast infections, says Gerbstadt. Recent studies suggest that thyme, cloves and even the essential oils from oranges are also effective fungicides.

Chamomile tea: is a cure for heartburn and can ease heartburn. It can ease digestive inflammation, says Bellis, steep 2 teaspoon of the herb in 10 ounce of very hot water for 20 minute.

Potatoes: cure for headache. The 37g of carbs in a medium potato can ease a tension headache by upping serotonin levels as long as, you keep the fat.

Biblical References

Psalm 7:1	Psalm 139:7-8	Ephesians 5:15
Exodus 23:25	Ephesians 4:30	John 3:34
Thessalonians 2:18	Colossians 1:16-17	Genesis 21:2-3
3 John 1:2	Matthew 7:13-14	Job 42:12
Isaiah 54:17	Luke 10:19	2 Corinthians 1:2-3
Jeremiah 31:29	Numbers 14:11-12	Matthew 28:30
Exodus 15:26	Ecclesiastes 3:1	Romans 8:28
Proverbs 18:21	Psalm 90:10	Jeremiah 29:11
Romans 4:17	John 14:1-3	Genesis 1:29
Psalm 103:2-3	Proverbs 4:7	Ezekiel 47:12
Philippians 4:13	Isaiah 26:3	1 Corinthians 3:16-17
James 4:7-8	Psalm 139:14	Leviticus 3:17
Proverbs 31:27-28	Matthew 7:7-8	Proverbs 22:6
Proverbs 22:19-21	Proverbs 13:24	Matthew 9:20-21
Ephesians 6:1-3	Matthew 6:33	Deuteronomy
2 Chronicles 7:14	Galatians 5:16	James 5:13-15
Philippians 4:9	Genesis 2:2	Philippians 4:19
Romans 12:1		

BIBLIOGRAPHY

Experience Life.Com, by Kristin Ohlson, June 2014.

www.en.wikipedia.org/wiki/jorge__cruise.

www.jorgecruse.com.

Good Housekeeping, pg. 64, May 2014.

www.droz.com.

(Channel 5, NBC World News).

www.josephprince.org/.../receiving-healing-with-faith-and-patience!

Experience Life.Com/pg. 64, June 2014.

Experience Life.com/pg. 87, October 2014.

www.yahoo.com/health.

www.drnorthrup.com.

www.womentowomen.com./memopauseperimenopause/ nutritional-relief-for   -hot-flashes/.

www.theherbalman.com

Experience Life, pg. 11, April 2014

www.preventionreaderdigest.com.

Schwartz, December 2012, Rudd Center for food policy on obesity.

ABOUT THE AUTHOR

The author, Ruby L Johnson, is a native of Bobo, Mississippi. She moved to Memphis, Tennessee in 1967. She received her bachelor's degree in Business Administration with a concentration in Accounting from Christian Brothers University. She received her master's degree in Business Administration with a concentration in Leadership from Belhaven University. She worked several jobs in the capacity of Staff Accountant and Account specialist. She is owner/chef of Ruby Lee's Specialty a catering service "Irresistible Flavors That Savor" and specializes in soul food, healthy eating and more. Ruby was the owner of Ruby's Sizzling Skillet, a soul food restaurant that specialized in healthy lifestyle. She coaches on lifestyle changes and how to maintain good health. She is a five time Half Marathon runner.

Ruby is an Ordained Minister of The New Olivet Worship Center, under the leadership of Rev. Dr. Kenneth T. Whalum, Jr. She accepted the call from God to preach on July 1, 2007 and was ordained on December 20, 2009. She is an active member of several of the 12-Plan Ministries of The New Olivet including Music, C.A.N.A. (Couples Achieving Newness Again), Healthy Congregation (Facilitator for The Cooking with Olives), and Mission (Prison Ministry).

She wrote this book because of her love for the people of God. I am so grateful to share this knowledge. Thank you in advance for purchasing this book. The author may be reached at the telephone number and email below.

901-826-2558
rubyjohnson1213@gmail.com

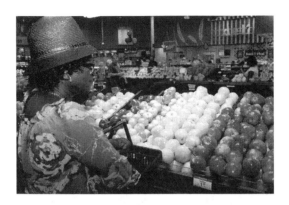

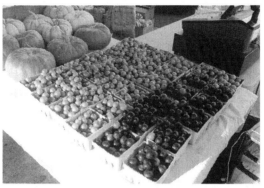

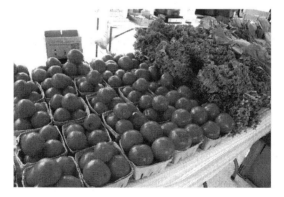

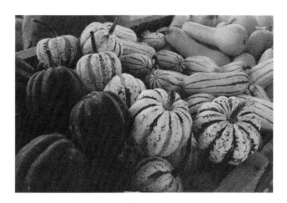

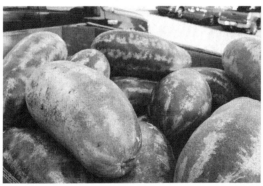

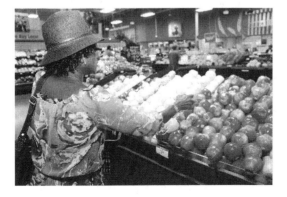

Made in the USA
Lexington, KY
16 July 2017